Praise for *Erotic Intelligence*

"*Erotic Intelligence* provides couples healing from the pain of sexual addiction with a road map to rewrite their sexual story, from one of betrayal, to one of healing, and finally to one of vibrant erotic sex."

—Stefanie Carnes, Ph.D., editor of
Mending a Shattered Heart: A Guide for Partners of Sex Addicts

"*Erotic Intelligence* celebrates recovery from sex addiction to healthy sexuality. It's a breath of fresh air."

—John Bradshaw, author of
Reclaiming Virtue

Erotic
Intelligence

Dear Nicole —
Best of luck in your recovery —
My you love well!

Alex

Erotic
Intelligence

Igniting Hot, Healthy Sex

While in Recovery from Sex Addiction

Alexandra Katehakis, MFT

Health Communications, Inc.
Deerfield Beach, Florida

www.hcibooks.com

Library of Congress Cataloging-in-Publication Data

Katehakis, Alexandra.
    Erotic intelligence : igniting hot, healthy sex after recovery from sex addiction /
Alexandra Katehakis.
        p. cm.
    Includes bibliographical references and index.
    ISBN-13: 978-0-7573-1437-7
    ISBN-10: 0-7573-1437-6
    1. Sex.   2. Sex addiction.   3. Intimacy (Psychology)   4. Sex (Psychology)
I. Title.
    HQ21.K2474 2010
    616.85'833—dc22

                                                                2009028856

Publisher: Health Communications, Inc.
        3201 S.W. 15th Street
        Deerfield Beach, FL 33442–8190

Cover design by Larissa Hise Henoch
Interior design and formatting by Lawna Patterson Oldfield

To all the men and women
in sexual recovery who have had
"the courage to change the
things I can . . ."

Contents

Foreword

"Will I ever have sex again?"

Understandably, this question is asked most often by sex addicts in the process of recovery. Layers of other queries lurk behind this primary question: "Will my partner ever respond sexually to me again?" "How will I know what to do to please my partner and myself?" "What is healthy sex, anyway?"

The either/or world of addiction recovery rules out having sex in the early stages, but what happens after that? Addicts still have a desire for sexual relations, and they are now recognizing a need to understand how they can have sex in healthy ways.

Most experts in the field of sex addiction have focused on understanding how it comes to be and how to stop the self-destruction. Alex Katehakis leads a new generation of sex addiction therapists helping recovering people claim a sexuality and intimacy that they've likely never had. In this honest and candid book, *Erotic Intelligence: Igniting Hot, Healthy Sex While in Recovery from Sex Addiction,* she uniquely addresses a multitude of ways to show how enjoying good sex and recovering from sex addiction can coexist.

Throughout the book, Alex explains how recovering addicts can "cut their own grooves" to support healthy behavior changes. She shows them how to build a coupleship that is mutually supportive and coaches them on being playful, sensual, and intimate, thus overturning the very premise on which sex addiction starts.

Alex applies her experience not only as a clinician but also as a supervisor of therapists who have completed the Certified Sex Addiction Therapist training program. Her concise, clear thinking continues to help dozens of professionals become stronger therapists. It is rare to have someone of her creative abilities also write masterfully about one of the biggest challenges in sex addiction recovery. I consider this book a great gift to all recovering addicts and their partners, who will benefit from its instruction, and an impressive, effective resource for those who help them.

Sit back and enjoy the ride toward a life of rewarding intimacy as you get answers to the questions you are asking. Yes, you can have sex again—in the healthy, supportive, sensuous ways you will discover within the pages of *Erotic Intelligence*.

—Dr. Patrick J. Carnes, author of
Out of the Shadows: Understanding Sexual Addiction

Acknowledgments

The idea for this book came to me in 2000 when I taught my first weeklong workshop on healthy sexuality at the Skyros Centre on the island of Skyros, Greece. Having worked with sex addicts for only three years and recently married, I was determined to understand the makings of eroticism and what it took to sustain a healthy sex life over time. The workshop participants came mainly from the UK and Ireland, and none of them identified as sexually addicted. However, they all had stories about guilt and shame in relation to their own sexuality, the topic of sex itself, and the messages they got from their culture.

The questions I constructed for that workshop were designed to open conversation among the participants—and open conversation they did! Every night at dinner, those in my workshop chatted about sex in great detail while participants in the mosaic or poetry classes sat slack-jawed, listening. A minor contagion took over, and soon the entire campus was animated and laughing—all talking openly about sex in healthy and bawdy ways.

Many thanks to the Skyros Centre for inviting me to teach that year, and thank you to the workshop participants for so generously revealing their unspoken secrets about their sexuality. You'll find many of the questions I conceived for that workshop in this book. A special thank-you to all the men who have been in my Monday night group over the years, specifically Mark T., Mark H., Glendon T., Van K., Howell T., John A., Howard B., Jimmie W., and Thomas M.

Although the names of the recovering addicts and their partners whose stories appear in this book have been changed for confidentiality, I thank every one of them. Without their honesty, courage, and generosity, writing this book wouldn't have been possible.

I have been influenced by many teachers, making this book a synthesis of ideas from all of them. I am deeply grateful to all of these people: To my mentor, John Cogswell, for teaching me to listen to the impulses in my body, helping me heal my psyche, leading me to my spirituality, and for inspiring me to become a therapist. To Patrick Carnes, noted psychologist and author, for fearlessly naming the problem of sexual addiction and for forging a path for people to heal their sexuality. To Roger Ford for his coaching and belief in me and to Larry Zucker for teaching me how to ask respectful questions. To Robert Weiss and Bill Owen for training me to be a first-rate sex addiction therapist. To David Schnarch for creating the Crucible Approach, a solid model for sex therapy. To Ruth Morehouse for her patience and clarity in supervising me in the Crucible Approach. And to those in the Wednesday morning group for their steady guidance.

To Noel Larson and the Zontain Women for their wisdom and willingness to dance. To Marion Soloman for helping me heal, encouraging me to write, and introducing me to Allan Schore. To Allan Schore and the Friday morning group for making my brain grow. To Aaron Alan and Jenner Bishop for contributing to the dating section, to Aaron for his feedback on the manuscript, and to

Chris Donaghue for his research assistance. My thanks to the women I lean on personally and professionally: Marta Stiles, Eugenia Buerklin, Julie Branca, Kathleen Gray, Margo Ingham, Tracy Masington, and Jess Sorci.

Many other people offered their guidance on how to write a book and get one published. I am grateful to these generous folks for their time and energy: To Caron Goode for shaping my ideas and helping me stay true to my beliefs and passion. To Angela Rinaldi, Jac Holzman, David Kramer, Howard Sanders, and Jane Jelenko for their shrewd advice. To Nancy Sobel for introducing me to Gary Seidler and to Gary for recognizing a need for this book and putting it into motion. To Christine Goodreau and Mike Ellison for inspiring the cover art. To Rosemary Marks-Carr and Adrian Carr for their filmmaking and photographic talents, and a special thank you to Wendy Maltz for her honesty. To Steve Delugah and Stefanie Carnes for reading the manuscript and for their valuable input.

To my editor, Barbara McNichol, for her extraordinary talent in bringing my voice and ideas to life. To Allison Janse, my editor at Health Communications, Inc. (HCI), for taking the baton and running it over the finish line. To Kim Weiss for her coaching and publicity skills, and all the others at HCI who put their talents into bringing this book to fruition.

I am constantly grateful to my parents, Sophocles Katehakis and Virginia Hardaway, for their steadfast love and for never giving up on me. To my sister, Nune Richards, for creating a beautiful space for me to do my work and for others to heal in. To the rest of my family for their love and support. And finally, to my husband, Douglas Evans, the love of my life, for walking side by side with me up the mountain, teaching me what it means to be intimate, and challenging me to love more deeply every day.

Introduction

Recovering sex addicts are the most courageous people I know. In assisting people through their recovery process, I have seen them recognize themselves as good rather than shameful or bad. I have witnessed them restore their sense of dignity and rightful place in the world. And I applaud them loudly.

Yet recovering sex addicts, their partners, and therapists frequently express the need for a practical guide for restoring their sexual lives. They want a plan for dating after recovery so they can experience lustful sex in the context of creating a joyful life together. And they want to build strong, spiritual, and supportive relationships with their partners.

This is exactly why I wrote *Erotic Intelligence*—to provide specific steps for sexually sober sex addicts and their partners to achieve these goals.

Who Does This Book Benefit?

If you're in a committed relationship, *Erotic Intelligence* explains how to reengage with your partner, get past the addiction awkwardness, and realize a sexual connection like you've never had before. You'll read first-person accounts of men and women in sexual recovery who have shared details of how their lives were damaged by addiction and then revitalized by clinically proven practices. Straight or gay, married or single, throughout this book you'll benefit from breakthrough thinking about what constitutes healthy sex after recovery from sexual addiction.

If you aren't in a committed relationship but would like to be in one, read this book as if you were. Imagine the kind of partner you would like to have and the kind of relationship you would like to build. Use the exercises to prepare for meeting the right person. If you are gay or lesbian, understand that all of these principles apply to same-sex relationships. Although certain sexual acts are performed differently depending on gender, you can easily translate the actions and related messages to your gender preference.

If you haven't already gone through recovery, *Erotic Intelligence* will show you what's in store should you commit to getting sexually sober. If you are newly in recovery or have reached a later stage of sexual recovery, I wholeheartedly congratulate you. Your courage to break free of sexually addictive behaviors has brought you to this point, which means you'll continue developing your sexual health and potential. As you will see, *Erotic Intelligence* assists you in discovering your own "erotic intelligence" so you can enjoy your unique sexuality through loving, connected—*and hot*—sex.

Your goal involves progressing through to healthy sex, then intimate sex, then erotic sex, and eventually sex as a spiritual act. Exciting, healthy sex comes from being *relational*, which means connecting deeply with yourself and your partner through your own recovery process. By developing an intimate connection to a significant other, highly erotic and spiritual sex can be yours. It stems from honest conversations about difficult topics that grow and strengthen your relationship. In this atmosphere, both you and your partner will feel safe to experience erotic sex. More than that, it will support your sobriety as well as your personal growth and development.

Reclaim What's Lost

I'm known as a leader in a new generation of clinicians who help recovering people reclaim what has been lost. I bring experience not only as a clinician but also as a supervisor of therapists who have completed the Certified Sex Addiction Therapist training program. After fourteen years as a therapist assisting men and women in sexual addiction recovery, I've learned to address their burning questions with success, as you'll discover throughout this book. Some key questions are:

- What do I do now that I'm sexually sober?
- Do my sexual fantasies have a place in my relationship?
- Does healthy sex mean boring sex?
- How can sex ever be exciting again?
- Will I ever be able to masturbate again?
- How do I talk to my partner about what I like sexually?
- How do I restore my sexuality as self-care, self-love, and connection to another versus a self-destructive act?

My experience has shown that you'll resolve these questions and feel the power of your sexuality when you understand how to develop more awareness—and more honesty—in your relationship. Achieving and sustaining sexual potential also means staying current with what's true about your changing body, sexuality, and sexual interests.

From there, you become committed to sharing those changes with your partner.

Commitment and Confidence

Understand that hot, healthy sex grows from a *mutual* commitment to your recovery. Your committed relationship empowers you to stay the course and maintain a strong focus when forming new behaviors. Toward that end, this book helps you learn to create a spiritual, transcendent experience—and create it in a healthy way. It's intended for you and your partner to release the pain of the negative story that sex addicts and their partners carry into early recovery. How? By following the guidelines inside these pages, you'll hone your own erotic intelligence and write a new story for your healthy sex life. As an even deeper, more significant benefit, you'll build confidence in your ability to achieve the intimacy you crave.

Confidence comes from being clear about who you are and what you want. You can express confidence even when it provokes fear or anxiety. And it develops, too, when you listen rather than react to your partner's feedback.

This book is not meant to give you license to act out sexually; rather, it's intended to lead you toward sexual healing. Therefore, as you read, if you feel like you're getting activated in ways that are uncomfortable or will trigger old behaviors, stop and take time to talk about what's going on with your partner, sponsor, or therapist.

Doing this will help you gain confidence because it leads to being clear about who you are and what you want. Realize that you can express confidence even when it provokes fear or anxiety. It develops, too, when you listen rather than react to your partner's feedback.

Know that both your relationship and confidence will evolve. As this book provides the steps to climb up the mountain, your commitment, skill, and joy become your truest rewards—ones to celebrate on your journey to the top.

Write Down Feelings, Thoughts, and Ideas

As you move through *Erotic Intelligence*, I suggest you keep a journal, notebook, or computer file in which you can write down any feelings, thoughts, and ideas you have as you complete the exercises. You'll find expressing them will move them from close inside you to a place of greater objectivity. Reflecting on your feelings in writing also helps you consider your choices more clearly while allowing you to set goals and move forward.

Let *Erotic Intelligence* illuminate your path to reclaiming your sexuality and the joy that goes with it. Enjoy the journey!

—Alexandra Katehakis

CHAPTER

1

The Dance of Intimacy and Sexuality

You count, I don't. I count, you don't.
Neither one of us count. I count, and
I'll try to make room for you.

—Virginia Satir (1916–1988)

At forty-three years old, Jay had never been in a long-term, committed sexual relationship. In fact, that's what brought him into recovery; he was scared that he would end up a lonely old man. After a solid year of working a program in Sex Addicts Anonymous (SAA), he was ready to find a serious relationship.

His first step toward preparing for an intimate relationship was finding ways to be kind to himself, to nurture himself. Jay started taking regular yoga classes, cleaned up and remodeled his house, spent time with other recovering people on the weekends, and created a social life he enjoyed. He had learned through his relationships in the program that he could be a good friend, loyal and trustworthy. He realized that his relationships with others and his family had meaning to him, that he "counted" to others. He felt more creative both at work and at home, even designing a beautiful backyard garden.

Jay was learning to "dance" intimately with himself and, in the process, preparing to be in a relationship with another. At this point, having a partner to "dance" with would be a strong addition to fulfilling his life. More important, it would represent a critical shift away from believing he needed someone to (presumably) make him feel good, share a social life, or clean up his house.

What Is Intimacy?

As a therapist working with clients recovering from sexually addictive behaviors, I've noticed how scared people are to approach having sex again after treatment. Often they have lost touch with themselves. Clearly, one of the most difficult things for people in recovery from sex addiction is discovering what intimacy really means.

If you're in that situation, *Erotic Intelligence* will guide you through reorienting your sexuality toward a richer, fulfilling experience with yourself and especially with a partner. It's meant to help you learn to "dance"—whether it's going with the flow in a relationship or exploring your own sexuality as a single person or both.

Throughout this book, the term "intimacy" refers to your ability to be close and have a deep, honest rapport with another person. The term "sexuality" refers to your capacity for sexual feelings. More than that, the concepts provide the foundation on which you'll build, explore, and develop a healthy, erotic sex life.

The prospect of having an intimate relationship and healthy sex life may seem inviting to you, or it may seem daunting. Either is okay. Know that you have the courage to change because you've made it this far, proving you have resilience and staying power. Your journey also requires knowing that the dance of intimacy and sexuality changes music often. As soon as you find the rhythm within a relationship, you might need to adapt and shift. That's why you have this book in hand!

Four Cornerstones of Intimacy

People toss around the word "intimacy" euphemistically to mean sex, but it goes beyond experiencing the results of the sexual act. Rather, it's knowing who you are in relationship to another person as you grow and change together. Your commitment to living with intimacy allows you to confidently learn how to create deeper relationships.

Understanding the "Four Cornerstones of Intimacy" can help you conceptualize what it means to be truly intimate. They are:

Cornerstone No. 1: Self-knowledge

All relationships start with knowing and accepting yourself. What do you like and dislike? When do you become anxious or frightened? Where are your growth edges? When you are out of your comfort zone, do you want to play it safe? When you are out of your comfort zone, how can you create an environment that allows change? Knowing the answers about yourself—and accepting them as your truth—enables you to do the same for another. Self-knowledge is crucial, given that sober addicts often talk about losing themselves to their primary relationship.

ᴗᴇ̣ₗₗ-acceptance means that you know who you are and are comfortable with that knowledge at this stage of recovery. It means that you are able to take input from those closest to you and decide what is in your best interest. This is not about making unilateral decisions or being selfish, but about making intelligent choices. The challenge of self-acceptance means *you know who you are and take a stand for what's true for you in order to create change, even when it's uncomfortable.* An example of this is setting appropriate personal boundaries. You can think of your boundaries as your own personal limits. You define those limits to your partner by saying "yes" or "no" in such a way that protects and maintains your integrity. Once you know what you need, you and your partner will be free to grow and change into more solid adults.

Cornerstone No. 2: Comfort and Connection

Sex addicts often find and create families out of a need for comfort and connection. People who come from difficult family backgrounds commonly have a desire for normalcy. Yet setting up a family is easy, but maintaining, nurturing, and attending to a family require diligence and discipline—two traits sex addicts don't typically possess. However, by *building connections to yourself and others, you can develop the capacity to comfort your anxieties and connect to your partner without reacting to his or her feelings.*

Paradoxically, addicts might turn away from comfort and connection to seek sexual novelty and intensity, which seriously disrupts the family in the process. Then, if the sexual object gets too close, they may run again. Addicts often bounce from family life, where they tolerate minimal connection, rebound to their addictive behaviors, and then bounce back home. One man in my therapy group stated, "In my addiction, I wanted intimacy everywhere but in my house."

Sex addicts who are single typically avoid connection altogether. Although they are seeking comfort and connection, they often report fears that being with one person will limit their options in life. Their inability to hold on to their individuality can have them acting in a reactionary way to another's needs, which may make them feel like they want to run away. Overcoming these fears, in part, involves *listening* to their partner's response rather than reacting to it.

Cornerstone No. 3: Responsibility with Discernment

Responsibility within intimacy requires discernment, which means *being assertive, speaking up for yourself, taking responsibility for your actions,* and *telling the truth,* even though it may be difficult for your partner to hear. To avoid conflict, most sex addicts find themselves accommodating their partners, meaning they adapt to what their partners want. They then "act out" their unexpressed feelings sexually as a way to feel a sense of power and control. Deciding to avoid conflict becomes easier than dealing with interpersonal conflicts.

In recovery, you become assertive as you face conflict head-on. Specifically, you discern the difference between saying things that are mean and hurtful and stating the truth about your preferences. An old adage states that addicts would rather ask for forgiveness than permission. But consider this: In a healthy relationship, people don't avoid conflict. They show responsibility by being direct and assertive about what they want and need. They choose to be accountable for their feelings and whereabouts.

As a recovering addict, you might use another adage that advocates you "stay on your side of the street." That requires *taking responsibility for your part in your interactions in healthy ways* on the way to reaching your goals.

Cornerstone No. 4: Empathy with Emotion

Empathy is your ability to recognize, feel, or experience another person's thoughts and moods. Reading your partner's thoughts and moods accurately is essential to building intimacy. Sex addicts often find it difficult to have empathy for their partner's feelings. They don't accurately listen to their partner and can get defensive when their partner expresses hurt, anger, or upset. Why? Because they may feel shame in the face of another's pain and make inaccurate assumptions about themselves and the other person. So in recovery, your challenge is to listen accurately by focusing on what your partner is saying about his or her feelings without defense or judgment.

There are two types of empathy: emotional empathy and cognitive empathy. Emotional empathy involves a bodily based feeling in our hearts or guts in relation to another. We can read the experience of another as if we had it ourselves. For example, if we see someone stub a toe, we wince. If our partners delight in eating their favorite ice cream, we delight in their joy. If our children cry because they fought with their friends, we feel sad along with them.

The second type of empathy, cognitive empathy, arises out of how we think we are *supposed* to respond. Cognitive empathy does not have a bodily based feeling to it. Rather, it's an idea born out of what we know to be socially polite, kind, and thoughtful. For example, if you see your dentist after learning that his grandmother died the previous week, you would say something like, "I'm so sorry to hear about your grandmother's death." You convey this because you genuinely like your dentist and imagine him feeling sad. Therefore, you offer your condolences even though you may not feel sad yourself.

Four Cornerstones of Intimacy

Make a commitment to use these Four Cornerstones of Intimacy as your guide.

- **Self-knowledge:** You take a stand for what's really true for you, even when it's uncomfortable, in order to create change. You know who you are, and you allow space and respect for your partner to do the same.

- **Comfort and connection:** You develop the capacity to comfort your anxieties and connect without being in reaction to your partner's feelings.

- **Responsibility with discernment:** You are assertive, speak up for yourself, take responsibility for your actions, contribute to all interactions, and tell the truth even though it may be difficult for your partner to hear.

- **Empathy with emotion:** You use your emotional ability to recognize and feel another person's thoughts and moods.

The Need for Empathy in Your Relationships

Showing empathy in your relationships helps you be comfortable with another and even helps you anticipate someone else's needs. Can you empathize with how your partner feels? Can you understand and validate how those feelings affect him or her without making them about you and having a shame reaction?

You will look through an accurate empathic lens when you:

- Know who you are and take a stand for what's true for you
- Comfort your anxieties

• Stay connected to your partner without overreacting
• Take responsibility for your feelings.

In active addiction, sex addicts are often self-centered and not oriented to others' needs. That's why they rarely take into consideration their addiction's impact on the needs and feelings of other people. Yet in early recovery, you discovered that having compassion for yourself was important. Now, developing empathy for another is a key component for intimacy.

Going through disclosure with your partner—meaning you've been rigorously honest in your communications about your history in the presence of a professional—is essential in recovery. It's also a major step toward regaining your integrity and living without secrets or lies. In fact, what you went through in early recovery gave you a head start on empathy after making restitution to your partner.

If you haven't made a full disclosure to your partner, do it before going any further. It's crucial to ask for professional help from a qualified sex addiction therapist when going through the disclosure process. Doing so will rebuild trust in your relationship and foster everyone's safety and well-being. Alternatively, if you do not have a partner, write a letter to someone you've harmed with your behavior. Write it from the vantage point of the effect you had on that person, not a groveling "so sorry" approach. Doing this will help you to take responsibility for the choices you've made and practice having empathy for those you may have harmed.

Where Attachment Comes From

Developing intimacy-building skills resulting in attachments to others starts in infancy through bonding between a child and parent/caregiver. Attachment done well results in that baby growing to regulate emotions and manage behaviors; done poorly, it's the basis of disconnection and a likely predictor for forming sexually addictive behaviors. What bonding is necessary for nurturing a secure personality? For infants and children to bond with significant adults, they need eye contact, facial expressions, gestures, tone of voice, and touching, all of which are associated with powerful feelings like empathy and acceptance.[1] This bonding creates the neural circuitry for how the child will learn to connect with people, tasks, and emotions. Similarly, the imprint of sexual awareness on the infant is influenced by interactions among the infant, mother, and father. Later in life, this can affect the adult's attitudes toward sex.[2] The early attachment period sets up a child's ability to respond to and integrate all environmental stimuli. Through the primary caregiver's loving touch and responsiveness, a child learns to feel secure and experiences his or her body as a safe place to be. If there's excessive stress in the environment, it inhibits the child's brain from developing properly, hindering physical growth and the capacity to connect.

Eye contact, touch, empathy, and bonding help a child's heart, limbic system, and nervous system adapt to people and circumstances. This is one reason why the concept of "attachment" parenting has grown in the last twenty years and why learning self-regulation has emerged as a main task in childhood.

What Is Self-Regulation?

As children develop, they learn to *self-regulate*, which means they have the ability to be aware of, control, and monitor emotional reactions, impulses, and behavior. More specific, self-regulation is the ability to repair emotional distress, usually through taking control and renegotiating the environment. A child who can self-regulate is motivated to respond to life and willing to change what doesn't work. Typically, the self-regulation skills for a sex addict were impaired during childhood. Learning these skills later in life can empower them to be adaptable and respond in more positive ways.

Usually, sex addicts have limited ability to self-regulate their behavioral patterns. The most common source of such disruption is being emotionally disconnected from their families of origin for a long time. Thus, going through recovery involves learning new ways to cope with the world and change old behaviors. Those who go through recovery are relieved to feel unfrozen in time and be intimately present in meaningful relationships. The result? They grow up as a whole human being and stop acting out adolescent sexual behaviors.

How We Cope with the World

Depending on how we are wired for attachment in infancy, we develop different ways of coping with the world around us and relating to adults. Here are four general ways people learn to cope:

1. **Unhealthy passive coping skills** include escape, avoidance, chronic sexual fantasies, isolation, and withdrawal from others. Unhealthy passive coping can engender helplessness, hopelessness, obsession, anxiety, and/or depression. This unhealthy, non-relational set of skills is referred to as *auto-regulation*.

2. **Unhealthy active coping skills** can run the gamut from using substances like drugs and alcohol to engaging in process addictions such as sexual addiction. These behaviors include, but are not limited to, excessive masturbation, viewing pornography, patronizing strip clubs and sexual massage parlors, frequenting

sex clubs, hiring prostitutes, cruising restrooms, voyeurism, exhibitionism, and the like. The relationship is with the substance or the experience.

3. **Healthy passive coping skills** include solitary activities such as journaling, reading, meditation, and contemplation. Physical activities such as skiing, swimming, and hiking as well as high levels of creative expression such as composing music, writing, making art, and solving mathematical equations render a flow state in the brain. This healthy set of auto-regulatory skills is a form of *self-regulation*. These activities can be done alone or include other people.

4. **Active coping skills** include engaging or acting upon the environment, such as seeking support or solace from others and getting help to generate possible solutions. Active coping, another form of self-regulation, seeks control of the situation using productive methods to build resilience. Examples include going to 12-step meetings, asking your partner for a hug, reaching out to people in the program, forming friendships, and/or seeking comfort from friends and family. Getting comfort and support from relationships or other people is called *interactive regulation*.

Role of Attachment and Autonomy Growing Up

Successful infant attachment and continued bonding lead to establishing emotional pathways in the brain and body for intimacy. They form the basis of heartfelt qualities people feel when engaged with their partners. Children who have developed healthy personalities are comfortable striking out on their own, taking risks, experiencing the logical consequences, and soothing themselves. The more they explore, achieve, and succeed, the more secure and assured they tend to feel. The result? They grow up to be autonomous adults who are competent in their interactions and confident in their decisions. They are able to soothe their own anxieties.

Attachment feeds autonomy, therefore autonomous people seek the connection and comfort of attachment in their relationships. They represent the yin and yang of life, meaning the equal and opposite values of control and nurturing, power and virtue. They experience the human bonding process to grow into independence, capable of negotiating people and tasks.

Yet people don't live independently; they seek heart-to-heart relationships to know themselves at deep levels, thus developing the biochemistry for intimacy. Fortunately, those who didn't experience intimacy in a strong way can learn to ignite it by going through the steps outlined in the pages that follow.

Fostering Autonomy Within a Relationship

Autonomy within a relationship means being committed to making choices that foster togetherness while also discerning what's in one's own best interest. This process is called *differentiation*, which is the ability to maintain your separateness and identity while in close connection with others. It's also the balance between individuality and being together without depending on the other's approval or acceptance to function. Together, they are relaxed, not driven by fear of abandonment or, alternatively, by fear of being smothered and dependent.

Differentiated people can tolerate the shifting rhythms of closeness and distance without being threatened. They are flexible, meaning they have the ability not to overreact to a partner's upset. They can operate autonomously even though their partners may want them to do things their way. Differentiated people can also tolerate the tension inherent in every relationship. In contrast, addicts have to learn to soothe themselves so they can live with the tension and anxiety that accompanies loving their partners deeply. Paradoxically, they also have to reach out to people such as a sponsor or other group members in a program and ask for soothing from their partner when they need it. Turning to others for comfort is how we learn to soothe ourselves.

But let's be clear here on priorities. A person's first level of being intimate is with *oneself*. To be intimate—to love yourself and eventually another person—requires growing up. Growing up can be painful because it means grieving the loss of your sexually addictive behaviors. You have to be willing to give up your old ways to secure commitment with another. This means that you take a leap of faith and trust that your commitment will bring you more pleasure, in a different way, than your sexually compulsive behaviors did.

That's when the real work of intimacy begins.

Know that the relationship game is about you making you okay. Get real—no one is in your life to save your day. Your partner can love and support you. However, whatever goes wrong is up to *you* to fix. For example, you have to first identify and then change your fundamental responses that don't work in relationships, then you have to get uncomfortable. That's a radical change from what addicts typically do. They don't repair old disconnecting patterns; they replace their partners, and then they reenact their patterns again in new relationships.

Risk Taking Leads to a Healthy Dependency

So how about a change? Why not create a fabulous relationship while maintaining a clear sense of yourself in recovery? To create a healthy dependency, you need to take risks while connecting closely with the one you love. That means stating your preferences without blaming or shaming your partner or yourself. By making choices like these, you can honestly explore sexuality with each other to the depth of your hearts and spirits.

Remember, intimacy is finding new ways to know your partner, share struggles, ask for your needs to be met, be willing to change, and keep dreams alive. Your journey includes proceeding from healthy sex to intimate sex, and then to erotic sex—all while developing a spiritual base for your relationship. Don't lose sight of that in this stage of recovery.

Sexual energy between two people is a primal force composed of power (energy that moves toward another) and virtue (knowing the energy between the two is right). When the intention to come together is to experience attachment and autonomy, then these energies create a balance between two people. As Roy Grigg states in *The Tao of Relationships*, "Togetherness includes separateness. Separateness includes togetherness. Within each there is the other."[3]

Romantic Love Is a Primary Motivator

Sex involves different moods and varied purposes, one of which is romantic love—a primary motivation system that resides in the brain. Romantic love combines the drive for sex and the desire to build an attachment with another. This drive is a selection process through which we seek another person for the purpose of having sex. We are programmed genetically to do this.

Here's what happens. When we fall in love, our sex urges go into overdrive because the novelty increases the production of dopamine in the brain. That then stimulates the release of testosterone. So as the novelty wears off, we have to rely on different, more mature mechanisms to become sexually interested in our partner.

People have sex for many reasons, but ultimately, *how* we have sex is a reflection of how we grow and change throughout our life span. For most of us, the kind of sex we had in our twenties was driven by hormones and high levels of dopamine. We were seeking intensity and looking for the perfect mate. If we rely on this picture as a sexual ideal, then we may have problems with our sexuality in our thirties, forties, fifties, and sixties. Bodies, preferences, and interests change over time. If we don't explore our sexual changes with them, the sex act will become boring, rigid, and routine. As we age, sex is no longer driven by our biology but by our desire to define ourselves as sexual adults.

What Is Healthy Sex?

Because the goal in your recovery journey is to experience healthy sex, how is it defined and what does it mean to you? In my experience, most addicts hold an adolescent view of sex, meaning they frequently associate sex with intensity—the higher the better. Healthy sex does include intensity, but "intensity with connection" is where you're heading now.

As you experience in detail the characteristics involved in healthy sex throughout these chapters, keep in mind these key points:

• Healthy sex is not *secretive* or *shameful* to yourself or the other person.

- Healthy sex is not *abusive* in any way.
- Healthy sex is not used to ignore or escape your *feelings*.
- Healthy sex requires an *emotional connection* of some sort with the other person.
- Healthy sex is about love, respect, mutual caring, giving and receiving pleasure, and a desire to know yourself and your partner in a deeper way. Sex can be intense, but the afterglow and heat remain, not dissolving into the next rush. It's the simple pleasures that express or celebrate the love you share that will connect you over time.

What Sexual Health Involves

Experiencing healthy, erotic sex is where you want this journey to take you. But what will that eventually involve? Consider these actions that make up some aspects of sexual health:

- Talking about sex (the act) and sexuality (your capacity for sex)
- Exploring your sexual identity through the rules and culture you grew up with and through the culture we live in today
- Knowing the functions of the sexual anatomy for both genders
- Cultivating good self-care habits
- Accepting your body without shame
- Cautiously integrating masturbation and fantasy
- Focusing on positive sexuality
- Maintaining a sense of spirituality

The Dynamic Dance of Intimacy

Human beings have the unique capacity to be highly individual while simultaneously being part of a group or community. This paradox is part of living and working closely with others while tolerating the varying degrees of tension that naturally occur when together.[4] Intimacy, in part, includes being close to another person while tolerating the tension of being in relationship.

The closeness is not always tense, though. What you feel toward each other can be a highly comfortable connection that lets you value the closeness or the "heart bond" with each other. The term "heart bond" barely hints at the richness of a safe relationship in which you and a partner cherish each other. However, the nature of the relationship and the closeness it brings will inevitably create conflict. Relationships are not fairy tales but real-life, dynamic systems that force people to grow and change.

Every time you risk talking with your partner about your changing sexual preferences, you risk having to calm your nerves while your partner reacts with possible discomfort, which can be scary. However, your partner's discomfort should not stop you from giving voice to what is true for you. In addiction, sex addicts usually don't give voice. They are often not assertive, and will instead act out their resentment toward their partners by having sex outside of the relationship.

Yet, you are changing now, and through intimacy, you'll learn to tolerate your partner's response by not reacting to him or her. *Your new skill is listening with an open mind and heart and calming your own beating heart.* You notice that you're involved in a dynamic, ever-changing dance!

✓ Erotic Intelligence Checklist for Chapter 1

❏ Sexuality is your capacity for sexual feelings; intimacy is your ability to be close and have a deep, honest rapport with another person.

❏ A solid relationship requires the Four Cornerstones of Intimacy: self-knowledge, comfort and connection, responsibility with discernment, and empathy with emotion.

❏ Differentiation is the ability to maintain your separateness/identity while being in close connection with another.

2

Cutting New Grooves

Every man can, if he so desires,
become the sculptor of his own brain.

—Santiago Ramón y Cajal (1852–1934)

As a sexually sober person, you're striving to move toward intimacy using new tools of awareness. Chapter 1 revealed a solid foundation called the Four Cornerstones of Intimacy: self-knowledge, comfort and connection, responsibility with discernment, and empathy with emotion. This chapter helps you claim these qualities as personal values while you make fresh and better choices in relationship to yourself and with another person.

Your new behaviors—part of the healthy sex you want to experience—are changing from early to later recovery, meaning you're no longer only focused on staying sexually sober. Rather, in later recovery, you're becoming more able to connect, both with people in the program and in your primary love relationship.

Creating new behaviors that enhance your relationships require that you "cut new grooves" in your brain, like grooves that were once cut into old-fashioned phonograph records. No, grooves are not *literally* cut into a person's brain, but this image metaphorically describes how new behaviors will become second nature to you.

When you started the work of eliminating the personally destructive sexual behaviors that kept you from having your preferred life, you already took the first steps to "cutting new grooves." As you repeat new behavior patterns, you're laying down new neural circuitry between neurons, thus creating new networks. Scientifically, the process is known as neuroplasticity, which refers to the brain's ability to reorganize neural pathways based on new learning experiences.

People Can Change Brain Patterns

Scientists once believed that brain patterns were fixed and couldn't change past the age of seven, but they've since been proven wrong. More recent neuroscience has documented how people can learn new functions or skills to change their brain patterns, thus allowing personal growth to occur.

Think of how toddlers learn. They place full attention on interacting with a safe environment to acquire a new skill like walking. In the process, new pathways in the brain are being developed. Yet if parents yell at them or spank them, it disrupts this safe environment and puts them on alert. Their attention gets divided between an innate desire to learn and an imminent danger in their no-longer-safe environment.

Similarly, as a child, you sought control, pleasure, power, and connection, all of which caused the brain to program your needs as top priority. But if you didn't get your needs sufficiently met by your caregivers, you may have sought behaviors that made you feel good—that is, activities that activated the reward center of your brain. When we think about eating chocolate cake, driving a new car, or having sex, this reward center responds by releasing a chemical called dopamine, as mentioned in Chapter 1. This chemical excites the body into action when danger is present—something referred to as the fight-or-flight response.

Step back a moment and consider this point: *Sex addicts are not addicted to sex as much as they're addicted to the rush they get from the dopamine released in their brains.* This means that sex is not the problem; it's *the abuse of sex to get high* that's at fault. They've seen that the more novel and exciting the situation, the more dopamine gets released, and thus, the greater the rush.

Realize that in your recovery efforts from sex addiction, you've spent much time, effort, and energy changing the addiction impulses within your brain. You've stopped seeking the intensity that dopamine gives you. It's now time to start choosing strong foundations for intimacy by "cutting new grooves" and repatterning your behavior to create a new priority in your brain.

Ray and Kathy's Story

"Cutting new grooves" for intimacy was a task that Ray and Kathy, in their midforties, chose as their goal when they began couples therapy with me. Ray was an introverted physician in private family practice in suburban Los Angeles. He worked long hours and became addicted to cyberporn for stimulation. Kathy, a counselor at the local high school, busied herself raising their two children in addition to her work. The couple described themselves as "prudish" and strongly believed they had to maintain a serious image within their community.

Ray realized he had a problem when an employee walked into his office while he was viewing online porn. When he finally admitted he was jeopardizing his medical license with this kind of behavior, he sought help. After being in Sex Addicts Anonymous for six months and giving Kathy a full disclosure of his behaviors, it was clear Ray avoided intimacy with his wife.

Through personal therapy of her own, Kathy was facing her own intimacy issues. The couple began a path of sexual recovery together, seeking therapy to increase their sexual desires and closeness. His remorse about his sexual addiction left him feeling chronically guilty and left Kathy feeling betrayed and hurt. Over time, they both reported that these feelings were healing and receding, and they expressed a readiness to reconnect physically.

I explained that the Four Cornerstones of Intimacy—self-knowledge, comfort and connection, responsibility with discernment, and empathy with emotion—provided the basis for new intimacy. I asked them to consider these qualities going forward. Through discussion and prioritizing, as their first goal the couple chose developing a physical closeness. They first committed to touching each other through affectionate gestures, then holding hands and gentle stroking and hugging. Next, they spent time touching and embracing in the familiar setting of their bedroom.

Though it was difficult, Ray was willing to deal with his discomfort in reaching out and showing new forms of expressiveness. In fact, he realized he had two basic choices: to be direct and change or to stay stuck and potentially lose his marriage.

Kathy, on the other hand, had to address how she'd held back her sexual desire for fear of what Ray would think of her. She also had to work with her desire to forgive Ray and choose to trust him again.

Ray and Kathy started to rekindle their sensuality by getting to know each other again. They talked about the first cornerstone of intimacy: self-knowledge. Next, they had to establish comfort and connection. They created a safe environment by agreeing to honor each other and not take the other's reactions or limitations personally. This gave Ray room for the discomfort of being touched to diminish, and for Kathy to give voice to her conflicting fear due to feelings of betrayal. They faced these issues with confidence and gradually came together.

The Role of the Brain in Cutting New Grooves

All of the strategies we use to develop a richer relationship with ourselves have one goal in common: *to make new behavior patterns comfortable and familiar*. The good news is that familiar addictive patterns can disappear by training the brain to remember new behaviors. And, thanks to the brain's ability to change throughout our lifetime, our brains reshape themselves at any age.

We know that the people and situations we remember from our early years have had an emotional impact on us. At this stage, we can put this concept of emotional association to good use in reformatting our brain for new behaviors. For example, mild to moderate stress stimulates the brain, helping us learn and remember better. For that reason, Ray and Kathy chose to start with one specific task in a familiar setting. Ray did not get much physical affection from his mother growing up, so his nervous system was not used to being touched. In fact, being touched was a stressor to Ray's brain and body. He had to learn to tolerate touch to expand his capacity for it. Like his brain, his nervous system has plasticity, meaning that it, too, has the capacity to change. It was stressful for Kathy to admit to Ray that she would like to receive oral sex from him. She worried about what Ray would think of her or that he would compare her to the images he looked at in porn. Her challenge was to first stop judging herself for desiring pleasure then to calm herself down while she told him.

Science has revealed that intense levels of stress or chronic stressors damage the hippocampus, the part of the brain that remembers. That's why excess stress makes us forgetful. Doing too many activities at once—multitasking—diffuses attention, fatigues the brain, and adds stress. Intense stress can also result from prolonged arousal or anxiety, which floods our nervous systems and may cause shutting down or acting out sexually. In contrast, physical exercise brings oxygen to the brain. Walking, dancing, and all movement activities create new pathways in the brain while organizing, scheduling, and prioritizing focus memory.

Being in recovery requires that you use discernment to recognize the fine line between the stress that's required to change patterns and the stress of intensity that can tip you over into addiction.

Two Pleasure Systems

Scientists have established that sexual addiction occurs in the brain, not in a person's vital parts.[1] Despite negative consequences, the intense high that people seek when acting out sexually requires increasingly more stimulation over time. When an addiction has hijacked the dopamine system, the addict receives the pleasure of winning the race without the effort of running.[2] As the brain becomes sensitized to one level of experience, the addict then craves and seeks more pleasure because dopamine raises the tension from "I want it" to "I've got to have it."

Yet, there's a second system for satisfying pleasures—one that has a calming, fulfilling effect that's caused by the release of endorphins. Endorphins are meant to soothe under stress; they can dull pain and create feelings of euphoria. Sex addicts are keyed into both of these centers depending on their sexually addictive behaviors. They can ping-pong from excitation to euphoria, unable to stop and tolerate the quiet connection of intimacy.

As recovery progresses, a sober sex addict can use this principle for cutting new grooves—that is, for containing the impulse for seeking "the high" and choosing new goals for pleasure or fulfillment in a safe, enjoyable environment. This is a big step toward intimacy.

Feelings Are Real; Perceptions Are Not

When efforts are focused on cutting new grooves, previous behavioral urges can emerge. By remembering that feelings are real but not necessarily reality, you can monitor how you handle your behavioral choices and ultimately your moods.

Let me explain how this works. Sex addicts and partners of sex addicts often have difficulty regulating their feelings. This usually leads to distorted perceptions of reality due to early learning patterns in the brain and the body. Our personal experiences from early memories distort our perceptions. It doesn't matter whether an experience is positive or negative; our brains and bodies react according to our perceptions of situations and people. The closer we get to another, the more vulnerable we feel. The more vulnerable we feel, the more likely we are to forget about a process happening in our own minds and a different process happening in our relationship. This is the time for putting the Four Cornerstones of Intimacy into action. Remember, they include knowing who you are, comforting your anxieties, speaking up for yourself, and having empathy for the other person.

Managing your anxieties and changing your thinking is not new to you because it's been demanded by the program from the beginning. It facilitates how you change from a sexually addicted person to a recovering person living in integrity. Plus, when you manage your anxieties, there's room to have empathy for the other.

Role of the Heart in Intimacy

An intimate heart allows and recognizes vulnerability as the path to eroticism, and here's why: The emerging science of neurocardiology (science of the brain/heart connection) discovered that around 65 percent of heart cells are neurons like those found in the brain. Clearly, the neurons of the brain communicate with the heart. The brain informs the heart of its emotional state, and the heart responds.

The Institute of HeartMath has measured the effect of the heartbeat on the energy field of the human body and the body's organs. Scientists documented that the human heartbeat emits the most energy of all the human organs, even more than the brain. Indeed, the heart trains the brain. For example, we've known for many years that a mother's heartbeat profoundly influences the fetus's growth in her womb, and the same heartbeat can calm a crying infant. The mother and the baby have resonance, meaning that they vibrate emotionally with each other.

The heart also influences the body's hormonal communication and electromagnetic fields. Just like a mother and child, your heart and your partner's heart share resonance when you are physically close, when you touch, hug, or gaze into each other's eyes. Shared heart

Tips for Creating Strong Self-Relational Skills

Here are several tips to help you take the next step toward a sense of belonging and greater confidence. These early recovery coping skills will continue to serve you in the later stages of your recovery.

- Reach out to others and ask for help. You don't have to make decisions alone or deal with your feelings by yourself. Use your sponsor.
- Make program calls.
- Record experiences in a journal or diary.
- Pray and meditate.
- Use affirmations.
- Use positive self-talk.
- Exercise.
- Retrain shallow breathing.
- Track the impulses in your body and ask these questions in this order: *What am I feeling in my body? What do I need? What do I want?*

resonance calms and balances your brain, body, and other organs. When you are present with yourself—or when your heart is open to your partner—this is intimate sexuality.

Relationships Begin with You

Remember, your first relationship is to yourself. Start thinking about which new behaviors you want to accomplish as part of your later sobriety plan by using the Four Cornerstones of Intimacy.

For example, your initial goal might be to focus on the first cornerstone of intimacy: self-knowledge. You'll find that admitting your own shame, guilt, or anger can bring you ease instead of tension. Choose a comfortable environment in which to practice new behaviors. Using the Four Cornerstones of Intimacy supports further growth and can help to re-create the bonding process you missed in the early years.

You can also think about using a single intention that can be as simple as getting to work on time or as complex as getting sexually sober. The point is that the goals you choose to support your relationship with yourself are based on the single intention of sustaining the optimistic quality of recovery. In fact, this intention is the backdrop of every goal you set and each action you take. Consequently, in the later phases of recovery, you'll constantly find yourself asking questions like, "Is this choice supporting my single intention? Does my action promote a quality recovery? Am I using the Four Cornerstones of Intimacy to take a differentiated stance?"

As the first cornerstone asserts, knowing yourself well helps you relate to another person, which leads to engaging intimately. Answering these questions will provide ideas for setting up the relationship you want to create with yourself:

- Can I look into myself and like who I am? If not, what's missing?
- Can I envision who I am becoming? If not, what's in my way?
- Is intimacy one of my basic human needs?
- Am I aware of my internal feelings when in relationship with another?
- Do I recognize my desire for connection? Can I admit it to myself? Does shame arise when I do admit it? If so, how do I handle it?
- Do I feel empty, waiting to be fulfilled in intimacy?
- Can I list my emotional needs and transform them into goals for fulfillment?
- Can I communicate these needs I've identified to another?

Another way to assess your current quality of relationship to yourself is by reviewing the healthy coping skills you developed in early sobriety. Try to recognize an area for improvement. List your strengths and what you've learned about healthy coping and share them with your partner.

Implementing the following list will spark more ideas:

- Identify myself as a whole person who has addictive behaviors, but know that I am separate from the behaviors
- Establish self-esteem, believing in my ability to keep walking through the recovery process
- Learn to forgive my behaviors and myself
- Choose commitment to self-awareness
- Be willing to speak about my needs
- Find a supportive community and stay involved
- Learn to accept help and support from others within my community

- Establish the resilience skills noted in stage one
- Realize how the same skills for self-preservation can be redirected to recovery and reconnecting

Addictive Sex Versus Healthy Sex

As animals, human beings are designed to come together and procreate. Having intercourse isn't rocket science. Like puzzle pieces, our bodies fit together. However, the societal trend is to have long-term, committed, intimate, monogamous relationships. Humans were not necessarily well designed for this.

I believe a more modern feature for us humans is the *intimate experience*. For a sober sex addict, these intimate experiences initiate personal conversations about deeper connection and sensuality and build a new relationship from the Four Cornerstones of Intimacy. To build a similar new relationship with yourself, I suggest you pay rapt attention to your instincts and listen closely to your intuition, combining the strengths of your brain and your heart.

Moving from where you were to experiencing intimate sex and then to exploring your sexual potential starts with knowing what behaviors you'd like to change. The following chart reviews the shame-based behaviors that you are learning to transform into healthy relationship habits.

Table 2.1. Addictive Sex Versus Healthy Sex

Addictive Sex	Healthy Sex
Originates from a shame-based sexuality	Deepens a sense of self and embraces one's erotic, animal nature
Takes advantage of others	Is mutually respectful and honoring
Compromises one's integrity	Reinforces a congruent sense of self
Confuses intensity for intimacy	Recognizes vulnerability as the road to intimacy, intensity, and eroticism
Reenacts trauma and cements arousal patterns in the brain	Allows for exploration, making meaning of the sexual act, and "rewiring" of the brain
Requires a level of dissociation	Requires one to experience the feelings in one's body
Is organized around the past and future (i.e., euphoric recall and fantasy)	Demands the experience of the present moment and staying *relational*
Relies on self-loathing and self-destruction	Relies on self-love and nurturance
Seeks power and control	Seeks surrender and vulnerability
Is covert and manipulative	Is direct and requires risk taking
Serves to avoid feelings at all costs	Requires the willingness to feel deeply
Is fraudulent	Demands honesty and creates congruence

Table 2.1. Addictive Sex Versus Healthy Sex *(continued)*

Addictive Sex	Healthy Sex
Creates a tolerance that requires more stimulation	Requires self-confrontation for growth
Requires compartmentalization	Demands truth and authenticity
Is rigid and routine	Is joyous, a celebration of life, partnership, and one's spirituality
Is without meaning and devoid of eroticism or a spiritual connection	Creates meaning and embraces one's erotic self as a pathway to spirituality

Source: Adapted with permission from Don't Call It Love: Recovery from Sexual Addiction, *by Patrick J. Carnes, Ph.D. (New York: Bantam Books), Table 7-2, p. 225.*

A Far Cry from Where You Were

Becoming a sex addict often has its roots in childhood or adolescence and is usually linked to early traumatic experiences. These experiences can include benign neglect and emotional, physical, or sexual abuse. If children or young people feel shame about themselves or their emerging sexuality, or hold emotional residue from having been sexually tampered with, addictive sexual behavior may result. Feeling ashamed about sexual urges and desires can become a pattern as an adult, leading to a shame-based sexuality.

In my experience, sex addicts are often opportunistic; that is, they take advantage of others (including their partners) whenever possible. Sex addicts live a double life and tell lies to uphold it. Remember, addicts tend to repeatedly compromise their integrity and confuse intimacy with the intensity of the sexual high they receive from others.

Why? Because sex addicts are most likely reenacting arousal patterns from their early childhood trauma, further cementing those patterns in their brain. Sexually addictive behaviors were often routine, rigid, and mechanical because the addict required the sex act to be performed in a certain way in order to reach climax.

Addictive sex usually requires an ability to dissociate in order to follow through with acts that are often degrading and destructive. During sex with a partner, addicts may engage in the euphoria that comes with recalling past sexual experiences, labeled "euphoric recall." They may also fantasize about some future sexual exploit. What's the outcome of these activities? The sexual experience becomes an avoidance of connection with their partner and their own feelings in the present. Sex addiction therapists refer to this as *sexually acting out* in the relationship.

However, sex addicts in recovery take responsibility for what they think and how they see the world. Men and women alike in recovery report that this requires admitting when they were wrong, doing a reality check with their partners, or checking in with a sponsor or someone in the program. When addicts change their experiences, their brains change (as explained earlier in this chapter), and their perceptions also shift. That's why it's important to emphasize open-minded thinking as well as sharing thoughts and fears with your partner. When you do, you can advance toward exploring and achieving your sexual potential.

Toward Achieving Your Sexual Potential

The sexually sober addict has experienced sexual intensity and fantasy, but hasn't yet touched the erotic spirit of sexual union: a full sexual potential. Sexual addiction patterns can include exciting sexual positions and acts, but usually leave out integrity, authenticity, and connection. To explore sexual potential, the addict's objectification of the other without connection falls away. The sober addict perceives a partner as worthy of sharing the sexual caring. What are the limits of sexual desire? Can sexual activity fulfill a level of transcendence? Is peak sexual orgasm a communion with spiritual dimensions?

I believe the answer to the two last questions is "yes," but achieving such communion involves negotiating through uncomfortable spots, just like a jeep negotiates potholes on a bumpy road. Don't let that stop you. You've been through the worst, have grown in strength and commitment, and have the best ahead of you. *Welcome the tension as a gauge of your strength and an indication that you are growing* in the later stages of recovery.

Turn Up the Tension

Cutting new grooves to experience sexual potential means processing the tension that arises as a result of establishing new patterns, one step at a time. The third cornerstone, responsibility with discernment, reminds us that rigorous honesty is required in a relationship and creates a tension that is needed for great sex. This tension has a different timbre than that of living with the lies of sex addiction. It forces both people to grow up; it encourages the recovering addict to be assertive and the partner to step into his or her identity as a separate person. Having difficult conversations will lead you to form a solid friendship and forge deeply relational, powerful sex.

Also, without tension, there is no stretching to learn and achieve. When people come to couples' therapy with me, I don't mitigate the anxiety so they feel better when they leave. Rather, we gradually turn the heat up to start the growth process. If we turn it up too rapidly, they blow out of therapy. If we dissolve all of that anxiety, we have no stimulation for learning. Extending oneself into new sexual experiences means talking about it, willingly risking discomfort, and grappling with pain. You know how to do this. You've already negotiated this terrain in early recovery.

Through truth telling and sharing, people learn to trust others again. My observation of couples in therapy is that they are able to stay with the feelings in their bodies, their emotions, and the discomfort of telling their truth. It helps them form a new connection. And when they do, they find their personal pacing through their growth process.

Inherent Desire to Heal

When our bodies are injured or hurt, an inherent intelligence naturally moves us toward healing unless the organism is debilitated or ill. Being in a state of disarray causes us to want to get better and be healthier.

Consider this comparison. When somebody is hemorrhaging, the paramedics immediately put pressure on the wound to stop the bleeding. Applying pressure to an injury not only stops the bleeding, but it can have the effect of forcing the body to become stronger—creating a scab that heals into fresh new tissue. In a similar way, recovery therapy exerts pressure on addicts by forcing the accountability factor to stop the addictive behaviors. Once these behaviors are contained, people feel stable enough to begin to do the deeper trauma work.

You've been through the pressure and handled the healing. Now it's time to embrace your sexual potential by welcoming the tension and innate healing to build intimacy through healthy, erotic sex.

Further Defining Intimate Sex

Intimate sex means creating a space for closeness so you can see and be seen. Intimate sex requires the Four Cornerstones of Intimacy to be in play with emphasis on the fourth one, empathy with emotion, for your partner. No longer driven by the chemical high of falling in love or chasing orgasms, intimacy and love become choices. That means you're choosing your partner and relishing the deliciousness of being chosen. At this point, you put into practice the rituals of connection you have created together, like setting the stage for sex.

This is the time to invoke the senses by attending to personal grooming habits, using scents, and introducing tastes through food and drink. Flowers and a beautiful setting provide a feast for the eyes. You can create physical sensation through the choice of fabrics and touch.

With open eyes, you look deeply into each other's souls. Doing this creates a vulnerability that builds on the disclosures you've gone through and encourages a candor about who you really are. This process creates an intimate, sexual charge born of truth and sensuality that encourages you to stay in your body, to feel and share your array of feelings. In intimate sex, you no longer hide out through fantasizing about others or dissociating. You are fully present with yourself and your partner, preparing for your journey into the erotic.

Intimate sex is vulnerable. You surrender, meaning you relax into the close, personal, and cherished feelings so you can embrace your erotic, animal nature without shame. Intimate sex relies on self-love, nurturance, and the willingness to feel deeply. Your vulnerability is a path to intimacy and eroticism.

Most people, especially men, believe vulnerability means being weak, as if needing protection from attack. But it also means being open to experience and sensation. Vulnerability in intimate sexuality means being open to receiving and giving love from your heart. A vulnerable heart that's capable of genuineness becomes your strength. You trust enough to not need protection. You willingly risk everything to tell the truth and are rewarded with wonderful conversations with your partner. "Wonderful" doesn't mean easy, but truth telling creates a sustainable relationship with a solid foundation.

By now, you've completed a full disclosure of sexual acting-out behaviors with your partner, and your partner has faced the pain of betrayal. Telling the truth is harrowing, as is hearing it. Your courage to risk combined with your desire for integrity with yourself and your partner move you toward intimate sex. Embrace it! Enjoy it!

In Chapter 3, we will look at the process of intimacy as you develop self-awareness and manage a lifestyle that allows new choices for intimate sex.

✓ Erotic Intelligence Checklist for Chapter 2

❑ Cutting new grooves lets you begin to experience your sexual potential by processing the tension of establishing new patterns.

❑ Intimate sex relies on self-love, nurturance, and the willingness to feel deeply. Your vulnerability is a path to intimacy and eroticism.

❑ In intimate sex, you are fully present with yourself and your partner, preparing for your journey into the erotic.

CHAPTER

3

What's Love Got to Do with It?

Love is what we are born with.
Fear is what we have learned here.
The spiritual journey is the unlearning of
fear and the acceptance of love
back into our hearts.

—Marianne Williamson (1953–)

This chapter explains how we are wired for love, and yet how easily we can be hijacked into loving delusions. Love—as many have lived, dreamed, and romanticized it—isn't what we think. Actually, love isn't always what we feel either. Consider the following example.

Lily, an artist from Colorado, met another artist, Jason, at an art exhibit. They felt magnetized to each other. Fascinated by their immediate feelings of familiarity, they went for coffee, and then had a romantic dinner that resulted in a night of passionate sex. "It seems I've known Jason forever," Lily insisted. "He is my soul mate." In the meantime, Jason returned to his wife, children, art studio, and business in Phoenix. Although he enjoyed the romp with Lily, it was a onetime happening in his mind.

What chemistry made Lily feel as if she had known Jason forever? In 2000, researchers Andreas Bartels and Semir Zeki of University College in London scanned the brains of a group of people ranging in age from seventeen to thirty-seven years old who said they were deeply in love.[1] The scans revealed that romantic love that's visible in the brain area is also responsible for gut-level feelings and sensations of ecstasy. Naturally, not everyone takes the same actions in response to these feelings and sensations. Early childhood attachment experiences, family background, and trauma history influence what each individual does. In this example, Lily's brain said, "Go for it, Lily. He's the one." Lily, of course, needed a reality check on her perceptions, considering her history of going from one "cosmic" relationship to another. Yet she felt ready again to choose a companion, despite a short time frame and the absence of a courting ritual.

Three States of Love

Helen Fisher, researcher at Rutgers and author of *Why We Love: The Nature and Chemistry of Romantic Love*, has described these three states of love:

1. Lust, or sexual craving, that prepares us for mating
2. Romantic love that moves us to a stage of bonding for mate selection
3. Longer-term bond, which enables partners to commit over

time to rearing children. This stage includes feelings of calm and security[2]

These love states are independent of each other but can exist simultaneously. The consensus is that humans evolved to procreate, not to create happy, romantic relationships as fairy tales and stories in the media would lead us to believe. Yes, love is made up of chemistry, and during the romantic love phase, many brain hormones cause people to act in unusual ways and think obsessively. From this viewpoint, love is a chemical cascade that creates mood states.

However, our cultural and social upbringings also shape our sexual preferences and levels of gratification. Knowing that humans are wired for love enables a sober sex addict to develop a common-sense reality-check approach to intimacy. That's why the hot sex we experience in our twenties changes over time. Our hormones and other biochemical factors change; so does our relational attachment to sex and partners. As we age, we tend to relish the feelings of security first, then add the excitement that sex brings to the relationship.

Romance in the animal kingdom reminds us of how our love chemicals work. Following Helen Fisher's three stages of love, when levels of estrogen and testosterone rise when we are human adolescents, we start to search for a mate. Lust keeps us looking, spurring our sexual attraction to potential partners through the release of pheromones, visual attractiveness, and social conditioning. Romance rings true in our bodies as we become myopic about the partner who appears to be "the one." Having an ongoing sexual relationship— plus spending time conversing and caring—cements the pleasure-bonding chemistry. As a result, the foundation for intimacy grows.

Because sex addicts suffer from what Dr. Patrick Carnes calls a "courtship disorder," they often get stuck in that adolescent "lust" phase. The recovery process strives for moving beyond the temporary attraction of lust, working toward the "attachment" stage. Having this goal demonstrates a commitment to forming an enduring relationship. Real love endures through hardships and distractions because these hardships become a turning point toward maturity. How does this apply to you? Assuming you're in a relationship, you have chosen to turn toward yourself and your partner in building foundations for intimate sex. As you find deeper meanings for love and developing a mature strength, think about this wisdom that came from a Native American client: "The buffalo on the prairie endures the snowstorm not by turning his back to it, but by turning and facing it."

In recovery, your challenge is to make sexual choices that lead to creating a long-term bond with someone you love—as research about love, connection, and marriage has told us. For example, researchers at the University of Texas at Austin followed 168 couples who were married in 1981 through their years of marriage.[3] What did they find out? That the couples who romanticized their partners and were passionate with each other early on committed to marriage within months of their meeting. Those same couples had a higher rate of early separation through the years than those whose courtship took place slowly over time. Those who took longer to get to know each other became the better prospects for long-term marriages.

Difficulty or distress can make people fight for their relationship, which can lead them to intimate love. Indeed, couples who make it through the addiction recovery process can see qualities in each other they had never seen before. They come to a new level of respect for themselves and their partners. Indeed, seeing through the lens of respect can act as an aphrodisiac that creates an intensity of both lust and love for each other.

The Hormones of Love

It's natural that sober sex addicts need continued support as they ponder the questions of love's chemistry, the intensity of sexual highs, and the prevalence of intimacy as they mature. Why? Because the same chemical processes for addiction occur in the world of love. In her book *After the Affair*, Janis Abrahms Spring offers this insight:

> Sometimes you need to take something apart to rebuild it in a stronger, more lasting way. Jung wrote, "Seldom or never does a marriage develop into an individual relationship smoothly and without crisis. There is no birth of consciousness without pain." And, so it is with intimate relationships. We enter them blindly, often effortlessly, swept up with passion and an idealized perception of the partner, often cocky about our ability to keep things hot. Most of us are totally unprepared for what lies ahead and ignorant of what's required of us to last the course. We may think we know what it takes, but, oh, how naïve we are. The affair shocks us into reality. Fortunately, it also invites us to try again. . . . There's nothing glamorous about returning to an old, battered relationship and working to repair the damage. But after sharing so much history and struggling to come to terms with the unbeautiful about the two of you, you may now feel more connected, accepted and accepting than ever before. You are wiser with more clear-sighted vision of what your relationship can become. . . . This is a time to rebuild, to commit yourself to a lifetime of renewal, to allow yourself to feel hopeful about your future together. This is a time to channel your energy into creating something new, something better than what you had before.[4]

Questions about the hormones that color our perceptions and cause erotic and erratic behavior deserve answers. So what *is* love and what is its relationship to intimacy?

Love is experienced in at least two ways: (1) a bodily based state created through attachment to another person that allows us to recognize each other with a deep knowing that ignites and changes our brains, affects our moods, enlivens our minds, and steadies our bodily vibrations, and (2) a chemically based chain of emotional reactions that causes us to feel attracted, sexy, romantic, affectionate, and desirous. Sometimes we act on these emotions.

Choosing Mates in the Animal Kingdom

Although the concept of love in the animal kingdom is considered dubious by the scientific community, the concept of attraction is not. The mating and courtship rituals of animals form the basis for survival of any given species. For example, *National Geographic*'s Earthwatch Adventures describes the mating ritual of the male Nile crocodile as slapping his snout in the water, emitting a loud bellow, then squirting water out of his nostrils. Likewise, humans choose mates based on attraction, courtship, and mating rituals. What's the problem? Humans often confuse the most fleeting feelings of sexual lust with love.

Did you know that only 3 percent of mammals form families like humans? Here's one example from researchers at Emory University. Like a human, a prairie vole (a mouselike rodent) has receptors for the hormones of bonding. When prairie voles mate, the hormones oxytocin and vasopressin are released, forming a chemical bond. The brain's reward center experiences a rush of dopamine, ensuring their enjoyment and desire for sex with the same vole again. Humans experience this process also, resulting in feeling attached to their mate.[5]

The montane voles are like prairie voles except they *don't* have receptors for the attachment and pleasure hormones. When they mate, attachment bonds do not form, so their sexual behavior becomes the equivalent of one-night stands.[6]

Play, Attraction, and Reward

All mammals play, producing joy and other benefits for their young. Human babies love safe surprises. Playing peekaboo is an example of a safe surprise for a baby, as are other games that stimulate the brain to grow. Surprises happen due to the novelty of something unknown appearing in the baby's world. Adults need novelty, too, for ongoing development and to create arousal states. Arousal can occur when, for example, we try a new food, visit a new country, buy a new object, or try something new sexually. These experiences then create pleasure.

Another form of arousal can come from communication that's dynamically changing between two people because it creates novelty. For example, when you suggest something new to your partner, or when you reveal a new part of yourself, this creates a novel situation that can ignite arousal between the two of you. In Chapter 1 we discussed interactive regulation as a healthy way of reaching out to others to get your needs met. Here I suggest that interactive regulation naturally happens by way of ongoing adjustments you may not even be aware of that occur when you and your partner are communicating. When you're open to being vulnerable, hearing your partner, and seeing your partner as a sexual being, new information is signaled by your brains and bodies between the two of you about each other and about yourself. This new information can create a sense of ongoing novelty between the two of you that can create sexual attraction.

Roughhousing is a prominent type of play in childhood that adults tend to let go of. This kind of play between two adults can lead to sexual arousal because of a rush of dopamine in the brain. We start to see our partners in novel ways and desire them. Rough-and-tumble play can be particularly erotic; wrestling, tickling, having pillow fights, and chasing each other create a sense of excitement. In the aftermath of disclosure, though, couples tend to lose their sense of play. Fear temporarily eliminates it. As one partner told me, "Sex addiction throws all sense of play and desire for sex under the bus."

Being isolated has an effect on one's desire for play, too. Sex addicts and their partners often become isolated from each other. Addicts in the partnership, consumed with acting out, require isolation to organize and engage in their sexually compulsive behaviors. The partners are often distracted with the demands of life and stand aside, feeling alone and unconnected. In recovery, partners can sometimes feel more isolated because of the shame that accompanies telling friends and loved ones about the problem.

Play activates certain circuits in the brain for feelings of lightness and joy. The brain requires warmth and support in order to develop strong social bonds. Over time, females seem to remain more playful than males. As they age, males seem to equate play with dominance. Although humans start out as a playful species, few socially sanctioned forms of play exist for adults (besides dancing or telling jokes) that have them verbally jousting, laughing, and smiling.

Reactions associated with love are tied to our emotions during the stages of lust and romance. Visual stimuli, such as seeing a handsome man or a beautiful woman (in person and graphically) signal the brain to feel attraction. Males and females are attracted to different qualities in one another. When a man sees a beautiful woman, his emotions ride high and his logic disappears. In contrast, females are attracted to a companion who can provide and protect. Thus, when a woman sees an attractive man, she wants to know how he thinks and acts, and eventually how he will care for her.[7]

Similar dynamics are at work within gay and lesbian couples. Some lesbian women are more masculine and are looking for a partner who can raise children, while other lesbians may be looking for a female who will take care of them. I've worked with many lesbian couples, and almost always, I detect clear masculine/feminine energies within each couple. Gay males are sometimes fairly evenly matched and other times clearly split between masculine and feminine energies.

Women have larger limbic centers than men. These are the emotional networks in the brain that orient women toward caretaking roles like child rearing. Men with high testosterone are more likely to get divorced and have extramarital affairs; men with low testosterone levels are calmer and less aggressive, making them more likely to get married and stay married.[8]

Lust Versus Love

When lust spurs us on to seek attractive people with whom we might mate, brain researchers call it "brainless" and poets call it "romance." I characterize the search for love as "passion," an intense and enthusiastic desire. However, this intense desire interferes with the brain's signaling of neurons. So what's happening?

Any substance that interferes with signaling (including love chemistry) changes parts of how the mind operates. After all, the body and brain's effective, accurate use of their systems (including how they releases hormones) is crucial for human survival. As described in Chapter 1, when aroused or intensely stimulated, the brain releases dopamine, exciting the brain into making irrational decisions. People stimulated with dopamine can't sleep at night, think straight, or keep their lives organized. This effect certainly occurs when people are in their addictions—and in lust.

Sex addicts and other people who have unhealthy attachments can't handle either *duration* or *proximity* in their relationships. "Duration" means committing to intimacy over time, while "proximity" refers to nearness or closeness in relationship. So addicts might be able to handle a long-distance relationship for a long time but couldn't handle being up close and personal for a lengthy interval, even in marriage. Generally, these addicts leave the marriage or go outside of it because they don't feel as if their needs are being met. They make up stories about not being understood. They seek approval constantly from an outside source or need constant sexual release to modulate their mood and nervous system. Their excuses sound like this: "I did this because she wouldn't have sex with me. She stopped having sex with me a long time ago. I would try, but she wouldn't really do anything about it. This is why I did what I did."

But the real story concerns lack of assertiveness when they can't confront their partners directly because of their fears of rejection and abandonment. In general, sex addicts operate from the part of themselves that was victimized as children or young people, especially when they grew up in a household where their needs were never considered. Being victimized as a child can result in sex addicts becoming victimizers in adulthood. More than that, they run from the promise of true intimacy in their relationships, creating wedge after wedge because of their own insecurities.

In recovery, the trick is to understand that *novelty is created in the brain by connection, allowing you to move in close and stay there.* You're cutting new grooves (see Chapter 2), which means making different choices that can lead to feeling uncomfortable. However, these choices can repattern both your poor relationships and your addictive behaviors. An example of cutting a new groove is to gaze deeply into your partner's eyes. When you do that, your brain will begin to register a unique, fresh experience, and you'll be on your way to making a significant change.

In therapy, couples will often sit on the couch together and will talk to me about their partners as if they aren't there. Next, I ask them to turn and face each other and look into each other's eyes. A host of discomfort arises because it's a novel experience, yet they see the task through. That's how they're able to cut new grooves.

As a sexually sober person, you're required to do what is counterintuitive for successful repatterning to happen. For example, you can turn to your partner when you feel scared or anxious and tell him or her what you need. You'd say something like, "I need your help. I need to tell you what's going on. I'd like your advice. I need you to listen. I need you to be with me."

Remember, when you do this new behavior in a comfortable setting, you're likely to achieve your goal of connecting with each other in a new, meaningful way.

Reconnecting Behaviors

These seven tips for trying new behaviors will assist you in cutting new grooves and getting closer to your partner:

1. While watching television together, hold hands. Turn off the disruptive sounds during commercials and talk with each other, engaging your eyes.

2. Turn off the television altogether and spend an evening talking, planning a romantic getaway, listening to music, playing cards, or creating new rituals for romance.

3. Go for a walk or watch a sunset in silence, then share what you noticed with each other afterward.

4. When you come home after work or an evening out, hug your partner with a full-body, heart-to-heart hug. Take three deep breaths with each other. This activity regulates your nervous systems and brings your hearts into resonance—another example of interactive regulation. Kisses are nice but hugs plug you into each other, creating profound connection. Notice any feelings or discomfort that arise and then talk about them with your partner.

5. Repeat the hug in the morning when you meet in the kitchen for your first cup of coffee or to have breakfast together. Research shows that the female brain naturally releases oxytocin after a twenty-second hug. The embrace bonds the huggers and triggers the brain's trust circuits.

6. Spend fifteen minutes every night checking in with each other. Take turns talking about how you're feeling emotionally, physically, and spiritually. Ask for what you need up front,

saying something like, "I need you to listen, give advice, hold my hand, give me your opinion." Do not give feedback unless your partner requests it.

7. Tell your partner what one thing you did to honor the relationship today, from following through on a chore to something more meaningful. Each night, alternate giving each other a ten-minute massage. The receiver picks the area, such as feet, hands, face, or shoulders.

Commitment to Intimacy

In partnership, you can help each other regulate your nervous systems and grow into closer attachment. When you hug, sleep together, or use prolonged touch or steady gazing, you're sending and receiving energy and information about heart rate, hormones, and nervous systems. Let's take a look at how this works.

While lust, romantic love, and love with attachment are natural states, during your sexual addiction phase, you may have developed fears and discomfort about revealing yourself sexually to someone you know well. Or you may believe that you couldn't enjoy sex the way you'd like to with your partner. As a sexually sober person, be aware of this belief or feeling, acknowledge it, and be willing to follow through on an action that supports your commitment to intimacy.

For example, it's natural for men and women to be attracted to other people and enjoy "looking" at the opposite sex. In addiction, sex addicts often dissociate into fantasy and get triggered into engaging in sexual behaviors outside of their relationship. In recovery, the challenge is to allow these feelings to be. You can next act with sexual maturity by turning toward your partner and sharing something intimate. You could phone or write a love note or send a single red rose. By bringing home any ardor triggered by the other person to your partner, you're honoring the intimacy in your relationship.

Think of it this way: If you walk down the street and notice lovely gardens of roses, then decide to cut each beautiful flower there, you'd be standing in brambles, bleeding from the thorns, as you laden your arms with all the flowers you cut. Why not just look at one flower, notice its beauty, appreciate it, and return to your garden at home?

This analogy represents another form of self-regulation. Your goal in the later stages of recovery is to experience all of this beauty in a fun, exciting way with a committed partner. The abilities of you and your partner to regulate your impulses, refine your interactions, or stimulate your fantasies allow you to have fun with healthy lust. Using mindfulness techniques to help you be romantic with each other lets you trust each other again when discomfort arises.

At this point, you are:

- Mindful of the triggers that can lead you to relapse (which is why you go one step at a time)
- Connected to yourself by being rigorously honest with your feelings and beliefs
- Connected to your program and loved ones, so recovery is not just about you. Thinking of others minimizes your chance of relapse
- Accountable to others in recovery with whom you can take risks with in order to be more real, intimate, and authentic

What Is Intimate Sex?

Intimate sex requires risk taking, which has the following characteristics:

- It's about giving and receiving.
- It requires truth and authenticity.
- It thrives on your willingness to be uncomfortable in order to grow sexually.
- It demands the experience of staying present with the feelings in your body and with your partner while fully surrendering to the moment.
- It's relational and a joyous celebration of life, your partnership, and your spirituality.
- It dictates mutual respect, like saying "yes" and meaning it, or hearing "no," honoring it, and not taking it personally.
- It's the willingness to step out of your comfort zone in order to learn about yourself as well as your partner.
- It requires stretching and learning to reserve judgment when uncomfortable and confront limitations when they arise.

Tony and Grace's Story

Tony, at thirty-eight years of age, had a long history of avoiding women due to his relationship with his mother. She had always made him her confidant, inappropriately including him in intimate discussions about her relationship with his father. Tony's sexual addiction was characterized by a history of acting out sexually with prostitutes and viewing pornographic images of women dominating men.

Once Tony was sexually sober, he became sexually anorexic, meaning he put a lot of energy into avoiding sex as a way to feel powerful and have a sense of control in his life. Eventually he was ready to wade into the waters of dating. Clumsy at first, he never went out with anyone longer than a few months . . . until he met Grace, who was twenty-five. Grace piqued his interest.

At first they took it slow and didn't have sex for three months. They then kissed and touched, which gradually led to having oral sex. After dating for nine months and being sexual in this way, Tony and Grace moved to having intercourse. Initially, Tony was squeamish about it, feeling a little disgusted because he perceived that Grace always wanted something from him. In fact, he complained that Grace seemed needy. She wanted to see him more than he wanted to see her. She initiated sex more than he did. She wanted to talk to him about what she was dealing with in her life. In response, he thought she was immature and worried that she was too young for him. He wanted someone who was more of an adult and much less needy.

One day in therapy, Tony discovered that he never went to Grace with his needs. He never asked her to listen to his struggles with work and family or help around his apartment. Although they spent most of their time at Tony's apartment, he never invited her to shop for groceries.

Because Tony's mother was so emotionally inappropriate with him regarding his needs, he shut the door on having them. He didn't want to feel that female invasion again. Finally, he recognized that his fear of invasion kept him from loving and being loved. I reminded Tony of the Four Cornerstones of Intimacy and how he could choose to tolerate the tensions of getting closer to Grace.

Knowing the relationship had to either move forward or end, he decided to try a different behavior to make it work.

Tony reported that he spoke to Grace about his discovery over a two-week period, then they took a weekend trip together to meet his friends and family. Tony stated that when he talked to Grace about what was going on with him, she felt like a partner to him rather than a needy little girl. This helped him realize he had to move toward what was uncomfortable for him to change. He set a pace that he could handle.

Tony told me he and Grace enjoyed good sex on their weekend getaway. This was a huge step for him, given that he'd experienced sex as "gross, disgusting, and suffocating" at times. He enjoyed the physical pleasure, but intercourse itself still felt mechanical. We discerned together that he felt this way because he hadn't opened his heart to her completely—doing so was too scary. Staying in his body and striving to enjoy the pleasure was enough at this stage. Tony was able to maintain his erection and enjoy connecting with Grace. He even told her he loved her several times but still felt uncomfortable about it.

In fact, bringing up love during sex made him more nervous, so another behavior Tony wanted to stretch was talking lovingly and erotically with Grace. When he saw she was aroused by it, he enjoyed sharing that intimacy.

As Tony and I talked about his sexuality, he stated what it meant for him to admit to himself who he is sexually. This would require accepting himself *without judgment*. He grappled with this concept and is still not ready to unveil his proclivities to his girlfriend or sincerely tell her he loves her during sex. But he's willing to grow even more. For instance, he realizes that the only way to feel less mechanical and more involved with Grace is to admit that he loves her and to tell her this during sex.

Meanwhile, Grace was seeking answers to questions she was facing: Why did she want to have sex with Tony? Did she truly desire him? Did she want him to give her a sense of approval for being attractive? Was she tolerating the erotic talk because she thought it was what Tony needed, or did she really like it? Grace admitted clinging to Tony for reassurance and expressed interest in learning to desire him from a stable place. Taking responsibility for herself and her desire was key. After being together a year, they're both learning to face their issues and build a stronger bond.

Grow into Desiring Each Other

Everyone wants to "be desired" because being desired doesn't require vulnerability. If someone desires you, that puts you in the position of being in control. On the other hand, desiring another person takes work and time, especially when adversity has challenged the very fiber of a relationship. It requires vulnerability. That's why both parties in sexual recovery can sometimes feel afraid to initiate sex; they don't want to be rejected and diminished. Therefore, the challenge in recovery sex is to not take rejection personally, but to express fears and discuss sexual drives and preferences. *That means developing a clear picture of who you are and standing strong in your desires and choices.* Remember, the first cornerstone is self-knowledge, so take a stand for your truth, regardless of whether it makes you or your partner feel uncomfortable.

Sexual desire is a universal experience, yet no uniform standards exist for desire on its own. You could be sexually satiated or sexually anorexic. Like Tony, you may have a desire to connect with your partner through sex, or you may avoid it, finding it difficult to get closer sexually. Remember, your definition and expression of desire are uniquely yours. Without judgment or reservation, it's time to explore your own desire as part of rewriting your story.

Explore Your Sexual Desires

Use the following questions as a springboard into desire. Writing down the answers will help you clarify your thoughts and see them without confusion. Then you can make conscious decisions about having sex with a partner. Remember to include your answers in the new story you've started writing. Share your answers with your partner, too.

1. How do you define sexual desire? How does it feel? How does it look?

2. How do you express sexual desire?

3. Do you experience more sexual desire by yourself or with a partner?

4. Does your sexual desire for the other come out of a hankering or hunger for the other, or does it come out of your need to be needed, validated, or attractive? Which feels more emotionally adult to you?

5. How do you arouse sexual desire in yourself?

6. How do you let your partner know you are feeling desirable?

7. What do you like sexually?

8. How do you arouse sexual desire for your partner?

9. How do you make yourself understood in terms of your sexual needs?
10. What helps you feel loved?
11. When do you desire sex?
12. What are your motives for this desire? Emotional connection? Anxiety?

Desire Versus Stimulation

Why is it important to discuss sexual desires and preferences? Because it will assist your move into intimacy and openness. All decisions about how to approach your preferences for desire and arousal are "in the moment" and involve mutual willingness. Remember, you are endeavoring to be a differentiated person whose goals require staying truthful about your sexuality, your partner's sexuality, and your ability to manage the tension. You and your partner can do this one step at a time.

For example, many sex addicts report that they desired sex for sex's sake when in their addiction. As an addict, you may not have experienced any sense of desiring the other person you were sexual with if you didn't have a meaningful relationship with him or her. Consequently, sexual desire came from your brain's being triggered to release dopamine. In males, visual stimulation easily activates arousal. Women typically need auditory cues and a prospect of romance or relationship on the horizon. For these reasons, in early recovery, you were encouraged to ignore your arousal altogether as a way of understanding that sex wasn't your most important need.

Today, at this stage of your recovery, it's time to accept arousal, feel no shame over having or not having desire, and choose to enjoy sex with someone you consider to be a healthy person and part of your recovery. If you don't feel sexual desire initially with this person, slow down. Stay present through eye contact and engage your partner verbally and emotionally. When you do that, you'll find that desire will probably show up.

Carve New Neural Pathways

Remember the discussion about cutting new grooves in Chapter 2? We learned that new behaviors create new neural circuitry, which changes the patterns in our brains. Those new patterns then become second-nature behaviors, which makes the impossible become difficult and the difficult become easy. Over time, the easy actually becomes beautiful!

By your careful practice of being in the moment and engaging your partner, you're learning new patterns—cutting new grooves—for how to create sexual desire. Keep in mind these important points in establishing new behavior:

• Partners of recovering sex addicts, male or female, want to be desired but are sensitive to being used as sex objects.

• A woman's sexual desire must first come from her own differentiation and confidence about her sexuality. Her sexual desire is then activated by knowing that she's wanted by her partner. Continued bonding through touch, scent, and sound (what her partner whispers in her ear) leaves her feeling connected and loved. This produces arousal because she believes that her partner cares for her. When a woman feels cared for, she feels safe. This assurance allows her to be more uninhibited as her sexual nature comes forward.

• A man's sexual desire must also come from his own differentiation and confidence in himself. Free of shame, his sexual desire will also be activated by knowing that he's wanted by his partner. His partner's visual appearance and playful and seductive actions (such as being touched) often move him to be more connected and loving.

Table 3.1. Tips for Establishing Desire

Partner	Recovering Sex Addict
Establish an emotional connection.	Listen, be receptive, and respond actively to what turns your partner on.
Share your intimate desires.	Practice empathy, caring, listening, and touch.
Don't mistake your partner's sexual arousal as pressure to have sex.	Risk talking about what arouses your desire. Be mindful not to confuse sexual arousal with euphoric recall of past acting out.
Trust your instinct about whether your partner wants to "get off" or is working on his/her connection to you.	Learn to admire your partner's body in a related way by staying connected to him/her as a person, not just a body part.
Have fun without expectation in the moment.	Ask how and where your partner would like to be touched.
If sexual desire is low, work on making a meaningful connection allowing arousal to appear.	Explain how and where you like to be touched.
Don't deny parts of your sexuality or judge certain sexual acts.	Allow all of yourself to be seen, including your most vulnerable and animalistic self.

✓ Erotic Intelligence Checklist for Chapter 3

❑ Love isn't what we think or feel but a chemically based chain of emotional reactions. There are three different states: lust, romance, and attachment.

❑ In recovery, you strive to move beyond the temporary attraction of lust and work toward reaching the attachment stage. Having this goal demonstrates a commitment to forming an enduring relationship.

❑ Discussing sexual desires and preferences helps you stay truthful about what you're learning about your sexuality and your partner's, while managing the tension you feel.

4

Nourishment for Sumptuous Sex

Don't forget to love yourself.

—Søren Kierkegaard (1813–1855)

Each person makes new choices, defines goals, and sets schedules to put affirming steps into action. Each action becomes a conscious choice to move forward and become more familiar with you so that you'll ultimately be able to enjoy sumptuous sex.

Consider what's going on for these support group members:

- Caleb worried about the awkwardness of learning to date again. When should he disclose his sex addiction to a new person? How would the dialogue happen?
- Jon struggled with finding a supportive group of friends within the gay community, where sexual sobriety is atypical. As he

moved further into his recovery, gaining acceptance from a supportive community grew in his priorities.
• Rick, facing sixty, had no desire for immediate partnership. His desire was to make meaning of the life he had and the one he was currently creating. His future goal was to partner with someone in a healthy way for the first time.

As you work to change the patterns in your brain and behaviors, you're rewriting your life story with this intention: *to become an assertive adult who takes responsibility for your choices, actions, and consequences.* Chapter 2 defined the coping skills and behaviors you wish to achieve in the later stages of your recovery, while Chapter 3 addressed the nature and role of love itself. In this chapter, you'll focus on how to:

• Write a new story for sexual sobriety
• Focus your edge on personal development
• Celebrate yourself through self-care
• Reduce stress to increase sexual capacity
• Make healthy masturbation part of self-care
• Create new memory circuits for pleasure
• Build your support network

These topics address your relationship to yourself. Let's face it, the healthier your body, the better sex you'll have; the more mindful you become, the more present you can be; the more aware of your feelings and responses, the more watchful you will be to avoid becoming addicted again. Knowing yourself intimately makes you better aware of your feelings and clearer in your expressions now that you've moved through the old story of who you were as a sexual addict.

Remember, each choice and action is designed to feed your body, mind, and spirit with the most delicious cuisine, fulfilling in every respect.

Write a New Story for Sexual Sobriety

Throughout time, men and women found strength from their myths, the stories that explain how something in our world came to be. The characters in myths are gods, goddesses, or personalities who each represented a quality they desired to possess. For example, the Hawaiian goddess Pele represented the fire of the volcanoes. In Greek mythology, the goddess Athena symbolized wisdom, while the god Apollo represented light and truth. Today, the literary character Harry Potter has become a mythological hero. Harry represents truth and strength of character, which overcome the forces of darkness and destruction.

Mythological gods and goddesses can be used as motifs to represent human characteristics. The interests we have and the culture we live in influence the mythological characters we choose for ourselves. Today it's common for us to identify with well-known mythological characters or heroes played on TV or in the movies. For example, the hero of *Star Wars*, Luke Skywalker, has such distinctive values that he's easily recognized in American culture and could possibly be called a modern-day mythological god.

If you were to write the story of your early recovery from sexual addiction, you might say you gained strength by overcoming challenges, just as mythological heroes do. You challenged yourself by sticking with the program and making it to sexual sobriety. You might state that you came to see yourself as a person who knows how to change in the face of crisis. You have courageously completed a kind of hero's journey.

Now is the time to write the story of your later recovery and the journey ahead of you. What story would you like to craft about the sexual being you'd like to become? You can create a renewed story with your partner that unfolds through your writing. You'd describe what kind of sex you would like to have with your partner, what sensuality means to you, and so forth. The best way to start is to put your fingers to the keyboard or your pen to paper. Once you begin, stay connected to the writing until your mind is empty. Feel free to jot down thoughts, perspectives, and ideas that may arise as you move forward.

To begin, make a list of your strengths and skills. Be sure to include all the attributes you value about yourself. Need help creating this list? Review the following characteristics that people of different temperaments have.[1] (Most people identify with one, but it's also possible to identify with two or three of them.)

The Achiever: Self-assured; in control of the environment; a logical planner, leader, visionary, achiever; shows self-control; keeps track of self.

The Relater: Good team player, predictable, creates safety around self, values intimacy, uses time to advantage to observe people and build trust, avoids negative environments and people, easily influenced by others, loves the logical, values conversation, strives to complete tasks.

The Creator: Highly creative, helpful, relies on intuition to explore new situations, assesses outcomes, values spontaneity, influences others through sharing ideas and projects, values feedback, enjoys the limelight.

The Rock: Adaptable, strong-willed when needed, keeps to the middle ground, values harmony, is sensitive to stimulation, can self-regulate, likes having comfort for self and others, supports others, provides safety or balance to others, enjoys people and relationships.

Choose the qualities from this list that can mobilize your journey of intimacy with yourself, then create your own personal cluster of qualities. Remember, you're listing the *qualities you want to grow into as a sexually sober person.* Then choose a mythological character or a powerful animal that could represent your growth in your new life story. Writing your story through a mythological character allows whimsy and playfulness to inspire your muse, helping you to be bolder and more creative than you might be otherwise. Most of all, infuse fun into your story.

Focus Your Edge on Personal Development

During early recovery, your "sexual edge" (the point at which you got scared to try something new with your sexuality) was to eliminate self-destructive behaviors and agree to a period of celibacy. Now that you're in the later stages of recovery, you focus on personal development and intimate sexuality. On this edge, you're feeling and accepting discomfort as you try new activities and practice self-awareness with support from others. But you'll do them only with fun and pleasure in mind!

Holding the tension at the edge requires a willingness to move forward. Writing your personal story helps tremendously with this forward motion. You're honestly asking yourself what you want out of your sex life and what you'll do to achieve it. As you review your daily intake of things, think about and write down a few goals, then determine which actions to take immediately. Make these action steps part of your story. The chart below shows an example of how you could do this.

Table 4.1. Personal Development

Area of Life	Goal	Action Step One	Action Step Two	Action Step Three
Self-care	Get in shape, lose five pounds	Buy running shoes	Construct a meal plan	Run three times a week with a friend
Finances	Begin saving on a regular basis	Balance checkbook daily	Pay off debt	Open savings account and deposit biweekly
Spirituality	Define higher power	Buy books that appeal to me on this topic	Talk to friends about why they believe what they believe	Visit a place of worship of my choice

Completing a chart like this will help you understand how to handle taking risks with support from others. Here are four questions to consider as you begin writing. Explore each of them, then pick the behaviors or attitudes you noticed. You may find you'll want to incorporate them into your life story.

1. What are the thoughts and beliefs (the false I-dentities) that limit your life?

2. In what ways do you run away when you get anxious trying something new?
3. What will help you stop running away and sit still when you hit your edge?
4. What would help you have the courage to look inside, challenge your beliefs, and stay present with the anxiety, confusion, or discomfort you feel?
5. Who can support you and witness the courageous steps you are about to take?

Celebrate Yourself Through Self-Care

Will the new you, the sexually sober adult who's ready for intimacy, please stand up and identify yourself? As you view yourself in the mirror, can you see the confident one who is ready to nurture yourself?

Now is the time to celebrate yourself and feel more confident. How? By paying attention to what most addicts ignore—their physical health, appearance, and well-being.

Over the years, many sex addicts have told me they grew up in deprivation when it came to self-care. Although they may have had a roof over their heads, they didn't get the nurturing that comes from being disciplined to floss their teeth, eat nutritious food, tend to their clothing, make their beds, and so on. Without these, a person can harbor feelings of being shameful, undesirable, and not good enough.

So turn the tables and celebrate yourself—starting now. This means knowing you're entitled to eat well and tend to your bodily appearance, wardrobe, and living space. What areas do *you* need to address that will reduce shame and improve your confidence as a sexual person? Write them down as you set your goals.

Change requires diligence and discipline. Taking time for self-care is a discipline that's meant to be learned in childhood. In adulthood, it becomes a responsibility to oneself and to the ones we love, even though it isn't easy to change old patterns or begin new practices. In early recovery, you had to get in the habit of going to 12-step meetings, making phone calls to others in the program, keeping commitments to others, reading recovery books, and working on the steps. In later recovery, you'll continue to focus on all of the above plus take care of your health, repair your relationship, and define your sexuality from a new vantage point.

Self-care includes the following aspects:

Personal Hygiene. How is your personal hygiene, meaning do you look and smell clean, keep your nails trimmed, and take care of the small details as well as the large ones? Do you attend to your personal hygiene on a regular schedule? If you do not, set a regular schedule for taking showers, shaving, flossing, washing or cutting your hair, and other personal hygiene practices. Then follow your schedule. It's important.

Health. When was the last time you visited the dentist or had a physical exam? What other health concerns have you ignored? Set appointments immediately.

Diet. Are you eating well? Do you eat on the go or do you make a point of sitting down and mindfully eating your food? Are you distracted by wandering thoughts or television programs? Or are you fully savoring the nourishment you're giving your body? To supplement your diet, do you take vitamins every day?

Clothing. Do you pay attention to your appearance—not dress as a sexual object, but dress well to promote your comfort, ease, and confidence? Are your clothes clean, pressed, and professional-looking for work? What key items of clothing need to be replaced? Sort through your wardrobe and give or throw away what you haven't worn in two years. Dress for dignity, for your own self-worth, and for your confident comfort.

Cleanliness. How often do you wash your bedsheets, towels, and household items? Is every week to two weeks right for you? Do you need help keeping them clean? Inspect your environment for neatness and appropriate placement of items. Most of all, check for sanitation items. For example, are drains unclogged? Kitchen disposals kept clean? Garbage emptied regularly? Dirty dishes kept to a minimum? Cars cleaned inside and out?

Deep Breathing. When I ask clients to take a deep breath, mostly they suck air up into their chest, a movement that actually creates more stress. When under stress, we tend to breathe in shallow, rapid breaths high into the chest. A relaxed breath can go deep down into the abdomen. How we breathe reflects the tension we carry.

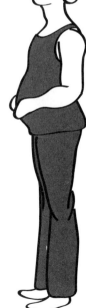

Breathing into your abdomen (the navel center) is an effective form of breathing for relieving stress and has excellent benefits. Deep abdominal breathing activates your metabolism, lowers your blood pressure, and increases vitality and energy. Do this breathing from a comfortable position—sitting, lying down, or standing. Expand your abdomen as you inhale, and then release the air gently with no force. Place your hand on your abdomen to help you focus.

Figure 4.1. Abdominal Breathing

Exercise. Do you work out with regularity? The body is designed to move, so if you sit at a desk all day, you need to move and get oxygen flowing. This is not just about looks, but about health and well-being. If you aren't feeling vital in your body, you won't feel good sexually. Find physical activities that include friends, your partner, or groups of people to motivate you to exercise and do it regularly. Did you know that exercise increases testosterone? It's the hormone that helps us feel desire and respond sexually.

Why Exercise Leads to Better Sex

Exercise benefits healthy sexuality so much that it should be on your to-do list every day. In addition, exercise creates more blood flow, relaxes the arteries, improves mood, and brightens any dire outlook. The main benefit is that it releases endorphins—and so do sexual activities.

Various types of exercise offer different benefits. Choose the type of exercise you prefer. Abdominal breathing revitalizes and relaxes; aerobic exercises are repetitive and rhythmic, requiring time to increase cardiovascular function and circulation.

If the intensity of aerobics doesn't suit you, try flexibility training. It improves your posture and movement ability. Also include yogic stretching or walking, along with abdominal breathing, as part of your regular actions.

Another choice is strength building to increase muscle tone and strengthen bones. Strength training also boosts your metabolism and cleanses the body. Be sure to include abdominal breathing with your strength training.

Exercise can also lead to better, more restful sleep, and both have been linked to a better sex life. Poor general health can lead to poor sexual function; keeping fit helps you sustain or enliven performance and satisfaction in the bedroom. A study at the University of Hong Kong showed that physical activity affects erectile dysfunction (ED) in men, which is the inability to produce and maintain an erection for the sexual satisfaction of both partners. Weight and low physical activity are the two key factors in creating ED. Men who did not exercise and were underweight were at risk for ED just as much as men who were obese.[2]

Women reap the exercise benefits too. One study by the University of Texas at Austin found that twenty minutes of moderate exercise enhanced genital response to sexual stimuli in women participants compared with no exercise at all.[3] In general, people who exercise regularly often feel better about themselves and more sexually desirable, and will likely have higher levels of satisfaction.

Even though you may have already addressed these self-care issues in early recovery, reviewing these components helps you focus your goals today. They lead to vibrant health and a balanced lifestyle, both contributing to intimate sex and strong relationships.

Reduce Stress to Increase Sexual Capacity

When your coping skills don't alleviate the perceived demands on you, what happens? You experience distress, which affects your sexual pleasure. While you were in addiction, that distress likely triggered you to act out sexually. However, in recovery, you're learning healthy coping mechanisms to handle similar stress—perhaps for the first time.

Stress and Hormones

Remember, stress *reduces* testosterone, which is the hormone that helps us feel desire and respond sexually. Cortisol, another hormone, can also have negative effects on sexual desire. Cortisol is called "the stress hormone" because it's released in higher levels when the body responds to a perceived threat or danger. When the danger is gone, the body is meant to return to normal functioning. Under chronic stress, cortisol will begin to have negative effects on the body, which can lead to blood flow moving away from the genitals. When stress turns to irritability or anxiety, then many men and women experience lowered sexual desire. Hormone-related issues like mood swings, sleep deprivation, or menses also affect our sex drives.

How can you monitor stressors and your responses? I suggest choosing activities designed to improve your health and well-being. Rather than take on more activity, it's best to structure a lifestyle around nutritious eating, movement, strengthening muscles, and endurance. These choices will help celebrate you and lead to sump-tuous sex.

Your Stress Checklist

The following stress checklist assists in understanding your responses to situations you experience. It's purposefully general, as symptoms of stress cross gender, culture, and age boundaries. Check the phrases that apply to you.

_____ Do you multitask, doing as much as possible in short time frames?

_____ Are you impatient with time delays or interruptions?

_____ Do you generally have a negative attitude when driving, complaining about others or conditions?

_____ Are you overly critical of coworkers or others familiar to you?

_____ Do you spread yourself too thin or volunteer for too much?

_____ Are you irritable most of the time?

_____ Do you have a tendency to feel guilty if you relax?

_____ Do you put off self-care for another day?

_____ Do you set unrealistic goals?

_____ Do you complain of being disorganized?

_____ Do you have few friends or a limited support network?

_____ Do you sleep lightly or is sleep interrupted at night?

_____ Are you constantly tired?

_____ Do you feel the need to share your drama with others?

_____ Do you worry a lot?

_____ Do you experience physical symptoms like headaches or high blood pressure?

_____ Do you experience holding your breath or shortness of breath?

_____ Do you experience moodiness?

If you checked six items or fewer on this list, you are managing your stress responses well. If you checked six to twelve items, your stress management skills are holding, but stress is taking a toll. If you checked more than twelve items on the stress symptoms, then stress is winning.

If stress is winning, you may be considered a "workaholic" and could benefit from Workaholics Anonymous (www.workaholics anonymous.org). You could also find a meditation program that works for you (www.learningmeditation.com).

Stress and Erectile Dysfunction

One potential side effect of stress on sexual capacity is erectile dysfunction (ED). ED has physical causes, and chronic dysfunction requires a visit to the urologist. However, ED can also result from psychological causes.

In my experience, men will report experiencing sex "in their heads" because they're worried about their performance. They're also focused on what their partner will think of them if they can't perform or provide pleasure. Often, because of shame, they don't even connect with their partner and don't allow themselves to focus on or receive pleasure in their bodies.

Yes, people focused on performance will have problems. Men who believe they have to live up to the myth that they're always ready with their erections will need to change their expectations. Women who have faked orgasm must look at their anxiety, too. Shallow breathing, self-consciousness, and anxiety can all be culprits for why women experience sexual dysfunction.

Your goal is to slow down and not be worried about results. Instead, you want to stay present in the process, breathe, and make close contact with your partner. It's important to consider whether you're touching your partner from the place of a confident adult or an anxious, shame-based adolescent.

Allow for your own pleasure and, with practice, these symptoms of anxiety will fade. Consider the first cornerstone, self-knowledge, and take a stand for what's true, even if it's uncomfortable. For example, if a man loses his erection, can he stay centered and not get lost in shame and self-judgment? Can he simply say, "You know, I was tired," or "I'm not really into it," or "I was really stressed out at work today"? As his partner, can you tolerate this without feeling bad about yourself or comparing yourself to his acting-out partners? Or if a woman is struggling, she doesn't have to desert herself by faking orgasm, therefore breaking the connection she has with her partner. Nor does she have to abandon the pleasure she is experiencing by putting pressure on her own performance. *The goal is for the self-aware person to feel comfortable enough to exercise self-acceptance while still being honest and authentic in the relationship.*

Derrick and June's Story

Derrick and June, a thirtyish couple with a two-year-old daughter, described their sex life as having little foreplay. He was a young attorney and she stayed home with their child. They called their degree of stress "normal." When they went to bed, they cuddled and touched, and at some point, one of them rolled on top of the other to have intercourse.

Derrick, who had chronic performance anxiety about keeping his erection, ejaculated quickly and then it was over. He hadn't worried about his performance when he was acting out sexually because he was hiring prostitutes and transacting sex for money. With June, though, he focused so much on whether he'd be able to please her that he couldn't settle himself down to enjoy the sexual act with her.

June had her difficulties too. She had an aversion to sex due to the chronic emotional abuse she had suffered at the hand of her mother, who was verbally sexually inappropriate with June as a kid. Consequently, their version of sex was super-avoidant, performance-based, and rapidly over with. Given that, we focused their therapy on dispelling the myths stemming from childhood conditioning. Their goal became discovering sensuality and learning a relaxed approach to having sex as adults.

In therapy, couples like Derrick and June ask themselves the following questions and discuss them with each other. I suggest you answer these questions, too, and share your responses with your partner or sponsor. If you do this with a partner, remember to use the Four Cornerstones of Intimacy to create a safe space for each other so that you can be honest and understanding. You can also use the answers to these questions as part of the new story you're writing:

- What were the messages you received from your family about sex and sexuality?
- What kind of role models did you have?
- Did you have any traumatic sexual experiences as a child or young person? If so, how did they impact your sexuality?
- How did you act out in your addiction?
- What do you consider to be "normal" sexuality?
- What do you know about what arouses you sexually?
- Where are you limited sexually?
- What scares you about sex or your own sexuality?
- What excites you about sex or your own sexuality?

After answering these questions, you'll see that your sexual patterns and preferences were forged through a variety of influential messages and experiences. These might have derived from family, church, early sexual experiences, television, movies, childhood abuse, and the like. The merger of these messages and experiences form what we call your sexual "arousal template." A distorted sexual arousal template could lead to sexually addictive behaviors. If your sexual arousal template created problems for you while in your addiction, challenge those patterns in recovery.

By honestly answering the above questions, you begin to form new sexual preferences, opening yourself to the possibilities of your sexual potential. This is the beginning of a new definition of who you are and what you like sexually. (If you didn't address this during your earlier recovery, I highly recommend reading *Facing the Shadow: Starting Sexual and Relationship Recovery* by Patrick Carnes, Ph.D.)

Make Healthy Masturbation Part of Self-Care

I compare healthy masturbation to shaving, brushing your teeth, or washing your hair. It's a natural part of self-care. Even if compulsive masturbation was part of your addiction, in time you may be able to make healthy masturbation part of your self-care and healthy sex life.

Many people in recovery think that masturbating means being unfaithful to their partner, especially if they chose masturbation over sex with their partner in their addiction. That misconception illustrates again why you should talk to your partner about your sexual needs, including your masturbation habits. You should also talk to your sponsor or therapist before you introduce masturbation back into your sexuality. Discussing your sexuality keeps the topic current in your relationship. In recovery, you simply don't want to have any secrets, lies, or surprises between you.

Gerald and Maggie's Story

Gerald, a cybersex addict, was married for twenty-two years when his wife, Maggie, discovered that he had been looking at porn on the computer for years, instead of having sex with her. Understandably, Maggie was angry and upset; she felt as betrayed as if he'd had an affair. In fact, Maggie was so angry, she wasn't interested in having sex with him at all and was also working through her own issue of having low libido.

Gerald understood and showed patience, but after ten months of celibacy, he desired some kind of sex life. After talking to his sponsor and group, he was encouraged, yet nervous, to make masturbation a healthy sexual behavior. Gerald was reticent about masturbating again because he didn't know if it would trigger him into following his old unhealthy behaviors. So he was instructed to limit his masturbation sessions to no more than two times a week. He was to do it in the privacy of his bathroom, stay with the sensations in his body, and stop if pornographic images began to come into his mind. Unlike in the past, in recovery, he said he stayed with the sensations in his body then eventually added the fantasy about having sex with his wife. I encouraged him to stick with that fantasy and see how he felt afterward.

Gerald understood that reintegrating masturbation would require paying attention to what he was thinking and feeling during masturbation and notice how he felt afterward. The sticking point with Gerald was telling Maggie about this plan. He loved her and was afraid to upset her. So Gerald turned to the third cornerstone, responsibility with discernment, and took a differentiated stance— that is, he would tolerate the tension this would bring between the two of them because he wanted something that might upset her. Neither person was wrong, and both had a right to their feelings. After all, they were two separate people.

Often, sex addicts feel like they don't have a right to get their needs met or express their feelings to their partners due to the pain they've inflicted on them. In effect, they put themselves in the emotional doghouse. In Gerald's case, he had to accept feeling okay about what he needed, talking about it, and respecting where he was in his sexual recovery. Maggie had to deal with the conundrum of not wanting sex with Gerald and the discomfort that his desire to explore his own sexuality in a healthy way presented to her. In effect, Gerald's move forced Maggie to look at her own sexual issues. She could no longer blame him for her issues, recognizing the amount of sexual sobriety time he had accumulated and the strength of his recovery program.

Sex addicts who have masturbated from the time they were kids usually report using masturbation to quell their anxiety. Often coming from rigidly disengaged or chaotic households, they discovered that masturbation made all their fears and upset go away. Yet, when it's not used compulsively, masturbation can be part of normal self-care, even providing a sense of renewal.

In his book *Great Sex*, Michael Castleman states, "Masturbation is our original sexuality. It's one of the first ways children learn to experience physical pleasure."[4] Indeed, masturbation is the best way to learn what turns you on sexually so you can communicate it to your partner.

Healthy masturbation feels good and doesn't require being concerned with pleasing your partner. Rather, you focus solely on your own pleasure by staying present with the sensations in your body, without sexual fantasy or euphoric recall of past unhealthy sexual experiences. Masturbating without having a goal in mind allows you to explore what's pleasurable. However, if compulsive masturbation posed problems for you in the past, you should not masturbate to avoid feelings such as anxiety and depression or use it when you feel sexually aroused. Instead, you may want to let the arousal arrive as you masturbate. *Healthy masturbation is not dissociative, a repetition of past trauma, or used to alter one's mood repeatedly.*

Masturbation can feel wonderful, but don't let it replace having sex with your partner. If this happens, or if you revert to past compulsive behaviors, stop and consult your therapist and sponsor, talk to your partner, and sort this out with others in your program before you resume.

Create New Memory Circuits for Pleasure

In later recovery, you are creating new memory circuits for happiness, love, intimacy, excitement, and novelty, as discussed in Chapter 2. You're now discovering that pleasuring these senses heightens your sexual enjoyment.

To increase your sensuality, remember to incorporate these three steps:

Step 1: Be present with yourself and your partner by paying attention to what you think, how you feel, and what cues your partner is giving you.

Step 2: Take time to consciously breathe. Deep breathing helps you stay present with your bodily sensations.

Step 3: Focus on staying connected to your partner and you'll experience pleasure with awareness.

Both men and women enjoy touching and being touched. Women are especially sensitive to touch because it allows them to relax and grow into arousal. Mutual touching releases the attachment hormone called oxytocin. Because men tend to rely on visual stimulation for arousal, they need to think about what to incorporate into a sensuality session, choosing something that empowers their ability to stay present and grow in the sensation of pleasure. A man may want to slow down and take time to look at his partner's eyes, face, hair, skin, and body parts that he finds sexually arousing. (Details about how to incorporate visual sexual arousal will be discussed in later chapters.) All this calls for writing into your story a scene for sensuality that brings forth your pleasuring muse. Creating the story increases your ability to visualize the scene; writing it down anchors the picture in your memory, cutting new grooves and reinforcing the images. As you do this, be mindful of not reverting to fantasy or euphoric recall that involves your previous sexual acting-out behaviors. If you're in a relationship, be sure to share what you visualize with your partner. You can even expand your experience by using gentle, soothing touch, caresses or massage, eye contact, and eye gazing.

Build Your Support Network

By now, you know that a large part of staying sexually sober is building a support network for yourself. Take time to add the kind of support you desire and the type of caring people you want to the story you're writing. Here are some examples:

Meditation Groups

James had difficulty being with people in general, so he joined a meditation group where he could be among people but without direct interaction. Joining a group for solitary meditation was his motivation to get out of the house and decompress after a crazy week. As he relaxed and increased his ability to be with people, his next step was to spend more time talking with group members and hearing their stories. He did a great job of listening. Because he found caring people in the group, he gave increasingly more of his time to the group's activities and felt more connected.

Friendly Pets

Research indicates that having a pet helps people enhance their social skills and overcome shyness. Marilyn had always been a pet lover, so she donated her time to the Humane Society in her community. As part of her recovery program, she adopted a greyhound that had retired from racing. Walking her dog every morning proved to be good exercise, and Marilyn found the early-morning dog walkers in her neighborhood friendly and talkative.

Positive Connections

You already know the benefits of having a personal support network. Your network might be simply for conversation or for moral support and accountability. Intimate, supportive conversation experienced in a healthy relationship opens your heart and reduces stress—both helpful in creating intimacy in your new story. Recruiting a special friend who will hold you accountable for your goals and action steps brings you confidence to achieve them.

Staying Present

Whether you choose deep breathing, meditation, optimistic self-talk, or journaling, learn to put your distress to rest. Say to yourself, "I am present, here and now, and I focus on [the task at hand] or [my lover, my friend]." Focusing in the present is a skill that moves intimate sex to a transcendent level. You can constantly practice this focus as you savor your food, listen to music, or gaze into your partner's eyes. You'll learn how to make sex more sumptuous every time.

✓ Erotic Intelligence Checklist for Chapter 4

❏ Monitor stress by making healthy lifestyle choices for better sex.

❏ Use healthy masturbation to give yourself a sense of renewal.

❏ Increase sensuality with these steps: be present with yourself and your partner, consciously breathe, and allow time for pleasuring yourself and your partner. Find support with caring people in the program.

5

Conscious Connection in Coupleship

Today stretches ahead of me,
waiting to be shaped. And here I am,
the sculptor who gets to do the shaping.

—Anonymous

In Chapter 3, you spent time becoming aware of and accepting your feelings, choices, and past behaviors. You're developing into a differentiated person who's in charge of your life while staying connected to others. You understand the saying, "To thine own self be true." In Chapter 4, you started writing your new life story. By this point, you've identified and listed your strengths, created goals for exploring new experiences, and developed an action plan. Your writing brings you clarity about your issues and also your solutions.

You've also begun to look explicitly at your sexuality and who you would like to become as a sexual being. You further developed scenes in your life story for building coupleship through intimacy. This involved two cornerstones of intimacy—comfort and connection, and empathy with emotion. Feeling whole and authentic, you arrive at the next step: *to establish or renegotiate coupleship.*

What Is Coupleship?

Coupleship is generally defined as a twosome; in this book, the term refers to two adults who decide to be in relationship with each other through commitment. Each chooses fidelity to move deeper into intimacy. Fidelity implies faithfulness, loyalty, and support to one's partner. In this case, it also refers to one's *sexual* partner. Making a long-term commitment to fidelity allows the time and space for creating a spiritual love that grows from your conversation, connection, and caring. Your desire to choose commitment speaks volumes about your sexually sober character.

It's possible you may have been in your addiction when you first entered into a relationship with your partner. Commonly, sex addicts weren't present in forming their partnerships, but they passively allowed them to happen. Many allowed decisions to be made for them, or they just went along with those of their prospective partner. Perhaps you even got married because others around you deemed it was the thing to do or you thought it would stop you from acting out sexually. Maybe you agreed to live with your boyfriend or girlfriend because he or she wanted to cohabitate more than you did. Perhaps you didn't feel attractive or lovable to the opposite sex and figured "someone" was better than "no one." You could have been afraid to say "no" to marriage at the time because you didn't have a clear sense of who you were. Maybe you entered into marriage to have an identity.

All of these immature reasons may have moved you to passively accept a partnership. But you've persevered and made it through the fogged lens of addiction to see coupleship clearly now. Presumably, you love your partner today and are committed to growing together. This time, you're making a choice about the kind of partner *you* want to be. And this time, you're choosing your partner because you know who you are and want a meaningful relationship *with this person*, not someone else.

Sharon and Gayle's Story

In the case of Sharon, an attorney, and Gayle, a university professor, commitment to each other had to be reinstated. They got together when they were twenty-five and twenty-three, respectively, and have lived together, built their careers, and had two children through Gayle's artificial insemination.

Sharon acted out sexually with other women throughout the course of their relationship and through both of Gayle's pregnancies. She finally hit a wall a few years ago and came clean about her occasional sexual affairs and endless emotional affairs. After Sharon's disclosure, both women had to rethink what they wanted.

Living in Connecticut as a same-sex couple, they could become legally married. Having been together twenty years with two teenagers, they seriously considered their options. Since they were in recovery, they both had to ask themselves difficult questions and share honest answers with each other. Gayle felt that Sharon was more forthcoming about who she was and what she wanted than ever before, while Sharon was relieved that Gayle was willing to tolerate conflict, knowing her childhood patterns had led her to avoid it in the past.

The ability to talk with each other and work out conflicts provides a step up on the path to intimacy. As noted in Chapter 3, we humans evolved to procreate—a basic drive that has us searching for a partner through the stages of lust and romance. Over time, the lust and romance that excites a single person becomes a sense of fulfillment when consciously connecting with another person.

Basic Requirements for Coupleship

Coupleship is as healthy as the individuals who enter into a commitment. Having strong "health" consists of the ability to:

- Heal your shame through self-awareness
- Forgive in order to move forward
- Take a risk in order to trust
- Shift from blame to responsibility and accountability

Before discussing what kind of partner you want to be in your relationship, let's address how to heal shame through self-awareness. After all, your own mental and emotional health is crucial to the success of your coupleship.

Self-Awareness and Healing Shame

Sexual shame lies at the heart of sex addiction. You probably developed negative thoughts and feelings about your sexuality if:

- You grew up in an environment in which sex was repressed, abused, overlooked, ignored, or deemed bad
- Sex was overly emphasized and your household was sexually charged
- You were taught that sex is dirty, bad, nasty, or the road to hell
- You repeatedly heard that sex is meaningless and that people use it to exchange neediness or get revenge

More accurately, self-awareness means the ability to identify your own needs and moods, and then be acutely aware of your responses. Remember, in early recovery, you analyzed the causes and patterns of your sexual addiction and learned to acknowledge your hijacked brain. Today, you're learning emotional responsiveness to others through participation in a 12-step program and creating a new role for yourself in coupleship. In reviewing how you've grown through your addiction, remember that using gratitude and forgiveness helps immensely.

Joe's Story

After Joe's parents divorced when he was three years old, his father became an absentee dad. As a result, Joe didn't learn how to be appropriately male around women. He was mostly passive with women and felt bad asserting himself because his mother was a feminist. She had grown up with a strict father and was determined to raise a son who respected women. In fact, she had repressed her own sexuality by not wanting men to look at her in sexual ways. Rather, she wanted men to value her solely for her intelligence. She had set good intentions with Joe because she wanted him to be kind and considerate instead of domineering and dictatorial.

However, this parenting style left Joe feeling as if he had to subjugate his assertiveness and natural male aggression around women to the point of feeling emasculated. He became sexually passive while feeling profoundly uncomfortable and anxious when regarding women sexually. His sexual outlets ranged from secretive masturbation, to pornography, to paying for sexual massage. Clearly, Joe was carrying his mother's sexual shame and repression.

Self-awareness enables you to change your focus to another task or topic. You can apply that to your sex life, too. As a sexually healthy person, you can discuss your negative or fearful thoughts with your partner or sponsor, then forgive those thoughts and move on. Here's an example.

Having worked through a recovery program, Jackson had gained insight and was becoming differentiated, meaning he was learning to be more self-assured and autonomous. One day, he and his wife, Kay, argued after she was reminded about the prostitutes he used to hire. He wrote about their argument and his tendency to go into a shame spiral, especially when Kay lost interest in sex. In the process, he examined his actions, accepted his shortcomings, and took responsibility for them. It gave him empathy for his wife's position on the issue. Later that week, he announced to his therapy group that he was finished with beating himself up and going into a shame spiral.

To know you can gain greater self-awareness, take a cue from Jackson and write your life story, reviewing the sex messages you heard within your family of origin. Perhaps your family members projected a cultural or religious overlay that distorted the meaning of sex. Remember, if you still hold shame and embarrassment about what arouses you and hide that from yourself and your partner, you will get stuck sexually. Were there sexual behaviors in your addiction that you wouldn't perform with a partner but would like to? If so, taking the risk to admit what you like sexually is a part of sexual recovery. For now, write into your story how you currently handle your thoughts or feelings of shame. Especially watch for shame that originally came from a parent or primary caregiver to creep into your awareness in this recovery stage.

Overall, your goal is to look at your sexually addictive behaviors in a new light. Have compassion for yourself as you review your character defects, shortcomings, and foibles. Attempt to understand why you developed them as a way to survive. Know that it's time for forgiveness by and for both parties to open your hearts and strengthen your relationship.

Process of Forgiveness Takes Time

For a couple to heal broken trust and fractured bonds, the forgiveness process needs room to breathe. It requires mutual support, attendance in therapy, and patience while you work through the steps of recovery. Recovery clearly takes time, especially for a couple. So hold steadfast to your commitments to support each other's processes as you work through your own program. Partners can help by reminding each other that the goal is forgiving, *not* forgetting, what happened.

In addition, know that forgiveness is not something you "should" do, but something that comes to you when you're ready. It arrives in stages, shows up differently for different people, and may never be complete. For example, glimmers of forgiveness may emerge after your disclosure discussion when both of you have begun to move through the grieving process.

Healing comes from remembering and talking about the destruction and pain you likely caused others by your behaviors. It also comes from continuing to move forward toward forgiveness and closure. Let's face it; you'll probably never forget the details of when you found out your husband was hiring prostitutes or learned about your wife's affair or were arrested for lewd conduct! And forgetting isn't necessary; forgiving is!

Recovery means forgiving yourself as you uncover past traumas and understand the patterns you've repeated over the years. When you're ready, you can explain these pains and make amends to the people you choose to, based on what you and your sponsor decide.

Eventually, you'll want to completely forgive yourself. Those you hurt the most will also need to make a conscious, even daily, effort to move on and freely forgive. That's when you're able to go forward and renegotiate your relationship with your partner. In time, the pain will recede. Remember to see the good, the true, and the beautiful in the world, your partner, your relationship, and yourself.

Self-Forgiveness Reminders

If you feel guilt for doing wrong or shame for being bad, or if you harbor resentment against your partner, forgiveness is needed for your recovery and to set the stage for sexual intimacy. Repeat these reminders daily to reinforce your resolve.

• I let go of my judgments of myself, knowing I was acting. unconsciously from what I knew and felt at the time. Today, I know better.

• The act of forgiveness changes me positively from the inside out.

• I make mistakes, own them, apologize, and start over with a greater understanding.

• I give myself permission to forgive my past mistakes.

• Forgiveness doesn't happen all at once; it comes in stages and may never feel complete.

• I am staying present and being aware of my choices.

• Forgiving myself prematurely can damage my health. I forgive only when I'm ready and listen to my heart about the right timing.

• Suffering does not make me a better person; pain doesn't create positive change; obsessing over the past doesn't ensure heart-break will not happen again.

• The opposite of forgiveness is resentment, and resentment will make me sick and keep me stuck. I release all resentment I feel.

Forgiveness is always about you for three reasons: (1) You are the only one who can make a conscious choice to forgive; (2) your choice to no longer focus on the hurt allows you to release it; and (3) forgiveness indicates you've reached an inner peace about the issue. That's how making the conscious choice to forgive allows you to move ahead with your life. How will you achieve that? You can start by *writing down how you perceive the task of forgiveness in coupleship*. For example, does forgiveness for you mean receiving an earnest apology from your partner? If so, are you ready to take it in? Do you owe an apology for any of your behaviors? If so, what are they? How can forgiveness help you in your situation?

Intimacy and Self-Nurturance

The word "intimacy" takes on a deeper meaning if you think of it as "into-me-see." This implies that, without first taking a hard look at yourself and having compassion for what you see, you cannot experience intimacy with another. Identifying where you came from and why you've done (and still do) certain things are essential building blocks for maintaining your recovery. Just as important is loving and nurturing yourself in the present.

Having compassion for yourself opens your heart to create intimacy with you and allows you to receive it from others. You'll also develop tolerance for others, opening you to receive caring, nurturing, empathy, compliments, hope, love, and much more from them. Think of it as true love for yourself. After all, self-love cannot be taken away and doesn't depend on others. And self-nurturing becomes lots of fun when you love yourself.

Let's look at two steps that lead to intimacy and self-nurturance: resolving past deprivation, and learning to appreciate your sexuality.

Resolving the Deprivations of Your Past

Think back to your childhood and make a list of what you felt deprived of or what was missing in your environment. How would you like to resolve those deprivations now? To give you ideas, look at these client situations and see how they're nurturing themselves today:

- Jennifer remembers her grandfather doled out the portions of Sunday supper, and she always ended up with the smallest portions of fried chicken and mashed potatoes, her favorite meal. To resolve this memory of deprivation, once a month Jennifer shares Sunday supper with her sisters, enjoying good company and healthy foods with them.
- Sam remembers his father taking him to his first sporting event where they had to sit in the "nosebleed" section because they were too poor to buy good seats. When Sam became successful as an adult, he bought tickets for sporting events and often bought courtside seats, taking his friends in the 12-step program with him.
- Marcos remembers he was banished to his room for "crimes" his brother made up, while his parents took his brother and sister to the movies. Today, he reserves Saturday afternoon for a pleasurable outing to the theater, and he invites a friend to ensure he doesn't withdraw into his aloneness.

What activities would enhance your confidence and self-nurturance? In your former life, beauty and sensuality were probably used to seduce others or ignored altogether due to the all-consuming demand of scheduling addictive behaviors. Yet life without beauty and sensuality becomes dull and dreary. *You can change that!*

Appreciating Sensuality

Take time to engage in your senses as a way to prepare for eroticism and sensuality. For example, go to an outdoor market and look at the produce or flowers, and touch, smell, and taste the offerings. Linger with the warmth of the sun on your face and body. Relish the color of the surrounding trees and flowers. Notice the sky's color and clarity. Train your self-awareness by staying present with sights, sounds, and smells as you go through your day. Be aware of the full-body arousal that happens when you're engaged sensually, and notice any difficulty you have staying present.

Then notice the tendency of the addicted mind to sexualize the arousal of sensuality and beauty instead of simply appreciating it and moving on. This, in effect, is how to apply the three-second rule that's learned in early recovery. What is that rule? You only have three seconds to notice how attractive a person is; then you must look away so you don't go into fantasy mode. *You notice the attraction to the beautiful, appreciate it as a recovering person, and move on.* Sexualizing what's beautiful and arousing can distract you from your feelings unless it occurs with someone you feel connected with.

Remember, healthy sexual arousal comes out of relaxation, openness, connection, and sensuality. It also comes out of being receptive to the present moment when your heart and senses are open. So make a mental note of all things that affect you sensually, then bring them into your living environment and let them change you. Become vigilant about watching your thoughts, choosing to stay present, nurturing yourself, and allowing your sensuality to arouse you. In doing so, you're on the road to experiencing intimate sexuality.

Strengthen Coupleship
Through Clear Communication

Know yourself and own your story—the first cornerstone of intimacy. If you don't know what you're feeling, you can't know what you need. If you don't know what you need, you won't know what you want. Depending on your partner to read your mind or figure things out for you puts you in a victim position. And what happens? Never saying what you need or want traps your partner into never getting things right. So know yourself. That way, you can communicate clearly.

I recommend applying these simple communication tools for rebuilding your life together:

• Stop and identify your feelings and needs in the moment.
• Make "I" instead of "you" statements about your partner. For example, say, "I feel abandoned when you travel" rather than "you make me feel abandoned when you travel."
• Take a moment to practice asking yourself what you're feeling. Close your eyes, take a deep breath into your belly, then check in with what you are noticing in your body. What are you feeling in this moment? Is there tension in your shoulders? Does your chest feel constricted or open? How does your belly feel? What are these bodily based feeling states telling you about how you feel?
• Then identify what you need based on that feeling state. When you are clear about your need, ask yourself what you want.
• State your current feeling clearly, its corresponding need, and what you want. For example, you might say, "I feel lonely and I need comfort. I want to talk to my good friend, so I'm going to call him/her and chat."

Using good communication based on knowing who you are leads to creating an interdependent, cohesive relationship. By standing on your own two feet and meeting each other from a place of honesty, you can be intimate in the truest sense. This means learning how to keep an eye on the good of the whole, not just on what each partner wants. It also means confronting who you are and looking at your part in any problem.

Matt and Jenny's Story

Shortly after they were married, Jenny realized that Matt's idea of a clean kitchen was different from hers, even though Matt was fairly tidy. She complained every time he left a dirty dish on the counter or a mess in the sink, accusing him of disrespect and considering her his maid. Once they talked about it, though, Jenny learned that Matt didn't hold these thoughts at all. He told her he was well aware of what she did around the house and thanked her for it. His tendency to leave a dish in the sink came from his hurrying out the door or thinking about matters at work.

Jenny reviewed her part in this dialogue to see how she was imposing her standards on Matt and causing friction between them. It was she who interpreted her own perfectionism as disrespect from her partner. Then she examined her options. She could continue to blame and shame Matt this way, or she could tell herself the truth.

Jenny knew that Matt would eventually pick up after himself, but not always on her timetable. She realized she could set her own standards, but she had to do so without resenting Matt. She also had to admit she did the cleaning, not because Matt was a slob, but because it made her feel in control during times she felt out of control. As a result of their communication, when she cleans, she knows why she's doing it and for whom.

So what does Matt and Jenny's situation have to do with sex? A lot! If you can't talk about what you need or feel in negotiating everyday life, then you won't be able to talk about erotic sex and what turns you on. Likewise, making assumptions can be damaging. Just as you can't assume what your partner is thinking when he or she leaves dishes in the sink, you can't assume what your partner likes or dislikes sexually. Assumptions like these can quickly dampen your sexual desire.

Communication Tips for Building Intimacy

• Shift your attitude from "me" to "us."

• Converse about feelings and stay aware of how you're listening.

• Learn to give suggestions without putting each other down.

• Listen without getting defensive or reacting to your partner's point of view.

• Discover what stimulates you and your partner and what doesn't. Communicate that in detail.

Stand in the Middle Ground Between Attachment and Autonomy

Recovery is filled with paradoxes. Here are two: (1) We're constantly reminded that it's a one-day-at-a-time process, yet we're asked to set goals for our future; (2) humans need connection and attachment, yet an important adult task is differentiation, or becoming autonomous.

These seeming contradictions exist everywhere. In recovery, negotiating them may make you feel as if you're living on the edge of uncertainty—but the edge is also where life becomes vital! *Too much constriction* creates rigidity while *no constraint* invites recklessness. In recovery, we look for the middle ground because that's where courage lives. It includes actions such as these:

- Ask your partner for comfort, such as a hug, when you need nurturance, and tolerate your feelings if you don't get it. If you aren't available to give a hug, explain why.
- Calm your anxieties in the face of your partner's upset and don't react, so that you can be there for him/her. If it's appropriate for you, try offering a hug.
- Set boundaries, or limits, when it comes to moving toward sex with each other. Talk about the pace that's comfortable for you. But don't use your discomfort as an excuse to avoid engaging sexually.
- Be curious about your sexual limitations. Take responsibility for why you don't want to try something new. Agree to examine the sexual act that makes you uncomfortable so that you can start a conscious conversation with your partner. Soothing your anxieties allows for the possibility of your sexual growth and development.
- Stand on your own two feet and ask for support from your partner when you need it.

While it's good to ask for what you need, you needn't rely on others to prop up your self-esteem. Remember, you have your own! Always dare to be your own person. You're internally strong and know who you are. That said, if communication breaks down between you and your partner, remember your part in creating this outcome. Don't take personally your partner's behaviors, statements, or moods. This refs to staying on *your* side of the street and not taking your partner's inventory. Don't blame, shame, or judge your partner's reactions; instead, have empathy for why he or she might be hurting.

Jasmine and Peter's Story

When Jasmine and Peter communicated what stimulated each of them, she was initially frightened to share what turned her on sexually. Peter was so angry about her affairs that he didn't want to know. Assuming she'd engaged in these acts with other men, he felt turned off and disinterested.

Jasmine took the leap to make eye contact with Peter during sex, all the while talking to him about her love for him and what she liked sexually. Peter felt her sincerity and chose to hear her suggestions without getting defensive or taking them as a put-down to his masculinity. The more Peter listened and responded to her suggestions, the more Jasmine felt seen, desired, and aroused. The more aroused she became, the more connected she felt to Peter. This aroused him further and encouraged him to love and pleasure her more.

A realistic view of intimate sex is that your sexual desire changes, and so does your partner's. These changes require your adaptation, both in behavior and how you communicate about them. What can you do? Take time to write excerpts of great conversations you've had (or want to have) with your partner about these topics into your story:

• What are the qualities you want in a mate?
• What do you consider to be normal sexuality? Does that excite or bore you?

- What scares you about intimate sex?
- What excites you about intimate sexual explorations?
- What would your ideal, realistic sexual relationship be like?
- What areas do you need to work on, and what is your commitment to do so?
- What amount, style, and type of sex do you prefer?

Remember Tony and his mother issues from Chapter 3? By confronting his fears and talking to his girlfriend, Grace, he realized that women didn't have any magical powers over him; they were just people. He became more comfortable saying he loved her while he was on top of her, thrusting and looking into her eyes. By doing this, he was more "in his body" and experienced fewer episodes of rapid ejaculation. While engaging in oral sex with Grace, he said that sex felt personal and not like a fetish as it did when he was in addiction. Tony successfully overcame his fear of getting this intimate. By facing his discomfort, he eventually felt closeness and connection with Grace more easily.

Do you relate in some way to any of the people whose stories appear in this chapter? What kind of partner do you want to be? To answer that, review the Four Cornerstones of Intimacy as guidelines for how you want to show up in your coupleship, then discuss your values, vision, and purpose for your coupleship with your partner.

Four Cornerstones and Intimate Sexuality

In Chapter 1, intimacy was described as being close to another to the point of comfortable connection. On this journey, intimacy in coupleship establishes the basis for a deeper connection involving erotic sex. Intimacy also requires moving toward and embracing the new learning, even if you are at the edge of discomfort.

Let's review the four cornerstones again in light of progressing to a new level.

Knowing Who You Are Requires Tolerance

The first cornerstone is self-knowledge, which means becoming more comfortable with yourself and your partner than you have been as you form a deep connection. The challenge of knowing who you are and accepting it means *you take a stand for what's really true for you, even when it's uncomfortable.* This level requires both parties to become more willing to move through issues or tolerate unpleasant situations so you can change and grow. Acceptance of who you are implies coming into alignment with your own values, choices, and solutions.

Connection Requires Trust and Risk

The second cornerstone of intimacy is comfort and connection, which means *you develop the capacity to comfort your anxieties and connect without reacting to your partner's feelings.* For a couple, this means establishing patterns for requesting what you need. These patterns can take the form of bonding rituals that help cut new grooves in the brain. It can also include meeting each other at the end of the day with a long hug, telling each other how you feel, discussing something you're upset about, and more.

Creating a trusting connection between the two of you lays a foundation to take sexual risks that can provoke feelings of anxiety. To grow and change, your sexuality requires *inviting the anxiety, tolerating the tension, and not reacting out of old patterns.*

Responsibility Requires Being Conscious and Present

In coupleship, the third cornerstone, responsibility with discernment, holds you both accountable for a certain level of maturity that reflects speaking up without meanness, managing your moods, and honoring your commitments. It also requires *being assertive, speaking up for yourself, taking responsibility for your actions, and telling the truth even though it may be difficult for your partner to hear.* You agree to remain present and conscious with each other.

The idea is to earn your trust by being trustworthy, attract your love by being loving, and show commitment through actions, not promises. At this point in your story together, there's no room for blame.

Empathy Requires Awareness of the Other

Empathy with emotion is the fourth cornerstone of intimacy. *It's your ability to recognize and experience another person's thoughts and moods.* Reading these accurately requires a differentiated stance and is essential to building intimacy. Remember that "differentiated" means you maintain your own identity while connecting with another.

Empathy can be enhanced by using another ability, "role taking," which means seeing the world from another's perspective. It requires putting your own feelings aside for a moment and stepping into your partner's shoes. Feel what it's been like for him or her to be in relationship with you, and what he or she is trying to communicate to you. As a good communicator, you will cultivate curiosity and learn to listen without interruption. Empathy is usually present in self-revelation, allowing partners to *finally* feel that they are seen, heard, and understood—as Justin and Brian's story reveals.

Justin and Brian's Story

For years, Brian tolerated Justin's lying, cheating, and bursting out in anger. Finally, he told Justin he felt emotionally battered and could no longer go on as they were in the relationship. Justin went into recovery and, through achieving one year of sexual sobriety, developed a degree of empathy for Brian.

For a long time, Justin had believed he was a good person because he was the primary breadwinner in the family. He also believed he wasn't hurting Brian by keeping secrets and telling himself, "What he doesn't know won't hurt him." In sobriety, Justin realized he'd told himself these lies in order to justify his actions. He saw how much Brian had sacrificed for ten years and the toll it had taken on his career and psyche.

Not only did Justin make amends, but he was also willing to change things, such as how he did business, the hours he stayed away from home, and the part of town they lived in. Listening to Brian, he was also feeling the pain of what his partner had lived through, understanding how Brian's self-esteem had been trampled on. Justin developed compassion for how isolated Brian had been from friends and family as a result of Justin's addiction. His empathy opened a door for Brian to grieve his losses and begin his own healing. Thus began their healing as a couple.

You base your ability to be present with your partner's feelings on your own ability to acknowledge and name your feelings. We call this "emotional" empathy as opposed to "cognitive" empathy. Typically addicts don't have much emotional empathy for others; they need to develop it.

How can you start gaining empathy? By staying in touch with your feelings and naming them on a daily basis. Also ask your partner what he or she is feeling as you make eye contact and notice what *you* feel in your body. Ask your partner questions about how the day went and so on. Listen to the answers and repeat them back to assure your partner you heard them accurately. This may seem stilted or contrived at first, but eventually you'll experience the benefits of this form of "active listening."

For example, when Mandy comes home at night, George makes an attempt to meet her at the door because he gets home first. Then they take a minute for a deep hug and a conversation like this:

George: "How was your day?"

Mandy: "Great! I finally got word that my project is a go. My meeting went well this afternoon, too. I feel pretty good."

George: "Wow! It sounds like you had a really good day. I'm proud of you."

Mandy: "Thank you. How about you? How was your day?"

George: "Ugh, it was long. I'm exhausted and frustrated."

Mandy: "I'm sorry. I hear that you're exhausted and frustrated. Is there anything you need from me?"

George: "No, not right now. I think the hug helped. I feel a little better."

Between George and Mandy, a little empathy goes a long way!

So far in this chapter, you've asked yourself what kind of partner you want to be and determined the values you wish to hold. Let's look at the purpose of your coupleship as a whole.

What Is the Purpose of Your Coupleship?

Although there's never an inappropriate time to discuss the purpose of your partnership, you'll probably have the most clarity to do so in the later stages of your recovery. The book *Mending a Shattered Heart*, edited by Stefanie Carnes, Ph.D., outlines these six stages for healing and recovery for couples:[1]

1. Developing/Pre-Discovery Stage
2. Crisis/Decision/Information Gathering Stage
3. Shock Stage
4. Grief/Ambivalence Stage
5. Repair Stage
6. Growth Stage

Most likely you're already in the repair or growth stage, but whatever stage you're in, be sure to answer this question: *What is the purpose of this coupleship I'm in?*

It's important that each of you take sufficient time to explicitly state why you are in the relationship. Both parties need to agree on a shared vision, a mutual purpose. If you can't agree, you should at least be able to comfortably live with the differences between your visions. Establishing that you're in agreement about what you want as a couple can give you a more solid foundation and provide a degree of security. However, if the two of you have extremely different reasons for being together, you may want to reconsider the relationship.

Certainly, stated purposes change throughout a relationship's life span. For example, a newlywed couple might answer by saying "to have fun and get to know each other." Another young couple might say "starting a family" is their purpose. A mature couple might say "to challenge our growth and development," while an older couple might say "continue exploring life together and solidifying our companionship into old age."

Consider the following questions about the nature and purpose of your own coupleship:

- Where are you in your marital life span, and where are you in your recovery stage?
- Do the stages line up? Chances are they don't, but whether or not they do, what does this mean for the relationship? If you're newly married and newly in recovery, what impact does this have on your relationship? After all, vows have been broken and dreams shattered. Perhaps you made assumptions about your partner you shouldn't have. Now is the time to get clear about where you're headed as a couple. If you're in the middle of your relationship and in early recovery, this usually puts major stress on the family. How does this change what you want for your lives? If you're in a long-term marriage and in the middle stages of recovery, this may be a good time to renegotiate the relationship, as you are both clearer now about what your needs are than you were in the early stages.
- What is the purpose of this relationship today?
- How do you define your own role in the relationship?
- What responsibilities are you agreeing to?
- What are you agreeing to as you continue into the next phase of this relationship?

Write down your answers to these questions and share them with your partner. If the answers you both give don't overlap, remember to use the tools of the Four Cornerstones of Intimacy as the basis for your communication. Take time to think about whether a disconnect truly exists between the two of you or if you're saying the same thing but not hearing each other. If you get into difficulty, consult others in your program and/or consider seeking couples therapy. Wading into the waters of intimacy and choosing to be in relationship is an adult task that requires you to stand in your integrity. No longer hiding out in the duplicity of addiction, you'll find your life becomes harmonious in that you say what you mean and mean what you say. As an adult, you don't avoid, couch your thoughts in vague words, or minimize what you want and need. Instead, you respect yourself and your partner while asking for what you want directly through conscious conversations. This process creates a closeness, or intimacy, that will transform you as you prepare to move more deeply into your sexuality.

✓ Erotic Intelligence Checklist for Chapter 5

❑ Coupleship is defined as two adults who choose to commit to fidelity in their relationship with each other. In coupleship, you make an active choice about the kind of partner you want to be. You choose your partner because you want that person, not someone else.

❑ For your coupleship to heal broken trust and fractured bonds, the forgiveness process needs time, patience, mutual support, and attendance in therapy while you work with recovery.

❑ Having honest conversations about your feelings, wants, and needs requires discipline, stretching to the edge, being nonjudgmental, and speaking consciously. To speak consciously means you talk about your experience using words that honestly communicate your thoughts and feelings without being hurtful to your partner. These explicit talks may set up resistance and discomfort, but they're crucial to establishing the intimacy you desire in coupleship.

6

Down to the Nitty-Gritty

The best and most beautiful things
in the world cannot be seen or even touched.
They must be felt with the heart.

—Helen Keller (1880–1968)

You're in the midst of writing a new story about who you are. Like a caterpillar's transformation into a butterfly, you have struggled through the cocoon of addiction to sobriety. Who are you becoming? How is your commitment to coupleship developing?

Let's dive further into the nitty-gritty of your conversations as you re-create your intimacy, sex life, sexual arousal, and eventually the erotic life you want.

What's New with You?

If you're the partner of a sexually addicted person, you've been through a major betrayal and have heard your partner disclose all of his or her sexual acting-out behaviors. You've experienced a recovery process and are moving toward forgiveness. If you are the sex addict, you've written a letter of atonement or restitution to your partner (who has accepted it), and you've gone through your own recovery.

So here you are—one or two years later—starting the conversation for your new life story as a couple. It includes sharing as well as renegotiation. If you're single, you may be dating for the first time as a sober person, or you may be tackling old issues with renewed commitment.

For example, a married client told me, "At dinner with friends the other night, my wife called me her 'old man' and I felt really weird."

"Have you talked about that with her?" I asked.

"No."

"Well, think about it. It's a good idea."

This man had difficulty making a conscious connection with his partner of ten years. Our culture upholds the notion that life is spontaneous and that events—sexual or not—just happen and needn't be talked about. But I encouraged him—and advise you—to bring up even small issues. Discussing them can help you both be more aware of your feelings and thoughts.

To talk any matter through explicitly is awkward for many people because they say it feels unnatural. If this feels unnatural, then making a date to have sex with your partner on a Saturday afternoon will feel artificial, too. However, making a date for sex is often required for people in long-term relationships. After all, people have busy lives, families, careers, and lots of other activities.

The conversation about being called "old man" raised questions for my client. Discussing it in the therapy group, we focused on the value of knowing where one stands in relation to a partner's expectations. It led to discussing these questions:

- What does it mean to be someone's "old man," girlfriend, partner, or boyfriend?
- Does such terminology imply specific expectations of you?
- What belief do you have for your partner in the role of "wife," "husband," or "partner"?
- When you're dating, how do you respond when you hear the word "boyfriend" or "girlfriend," and what does that role mean to you?

I suggest asking yourself these questions. Try on your roles, discuss your expectations with your partner, and listen from your heart. Share your interpretations and expectations of certain qualities of your roles. Having such conversations requires discipline, stretching to the edge, being nonjudgmental, and talking consciously. Overcome any resistance and investigate your own feelings further by writing down your answers to these questions:

- Why do these conversations make you nervous?
- Why do you avoid them?
- What do you have to do to comfort your anxieties and have these conversations anyway?

Your Inner, Middle, and Outer Circles

In early recovery, you listed all of your sexual acting-out behaviors that you are now committed to abstain from. This abstinence list, often referred to as the inner circle, is the list against which you measure your sobriety time in the program. That is, if you abstain from the listed behaviors for sixty days, then you have sixty days of sobriety. If you engage in the behaviors, you lose your time and start over again. This list may include, but is not limited to, viewing pornography in all forms, compulsive masturbation, visiting strip clubs, going to bathhouses, having anonymous sex, hiring prostitutes, and so forth. The list created is not negotiable; no matter where you are in your recovery process, you don't change it without consulting your sponsor, another sexually sober person in the program, or your therapist.

Next is your boundaries list, referred to as your middle circle. This list is made up of people, places, things, or states of being deemed hazardous to your recovery. It can include a coworker who stresses you out, a part of town you used to act out in, sex toys, sexual fantasy, or feelings of loneliness, boredom, anger, or tiredness. Engaging in these behaviors doesn't mean you have slipped, but it doesn't add to your recovery and could have you thinking about acting out again. This middle circle is more dynamic than the inner circle, which means you may add to it as you progress in your recovery. Again, consultation is required before making changes to this list.

Finally, your healthy list, your outer circle, includes behaviors that are life affirming and sexually healthy. In the early stages of recovery, your outer circle may list items like going to 12-step meetings, journaling, calling others in your program, going to therapy, exercising, eating well, and so forth. In later recovery, your outer circle now includes healthy sex with your partner. It can also include healthy masturbation—once you are clear about what this means for you and have discussed it with your consulting team.

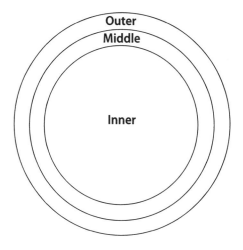

Figure 6.1. Example of Three-Circle Sexual Sobriety Plan

(For more information on how to create a comprehensive sobriety plan,
see the Sex Addicts Anonymous pamphlet *Three Circles*.)

Safety Planning for Partners

As a partner of a sex addict, take time to think about what you need in order to feel safe in the relationship. Often, partners report that they engaged in behaviors in early recovery that made them feel bad about themselves when they first learned about their husband's or wife's sexual acting-out behaviors. Understandably, partners will check e-mail accounts and phone records, listen to voice messages, or drive by the house of their spouse's affair partner trying to create a sense of safety and control. These behaviors can be destructive to one's self-esteem and are reactions to the trauma of having been betrayed.

As you heal your betrayal trauma and engage in healthier coping mechanisms such as reaching out to others for support, consider listing the behaviors that could lead you to diminishing your self-esteem.

This list might include (but is not limited to) feeling stressed out, waiting for your spouse's phone call, calling several times to check up on him/her, getting angry or jealous of your spouse's time away from home, and so on. When your instincts tell you something is wrong or when your anxiety increases, trust the feeling that comes up. However, remember to rely on your program and the healthy coping skills you have to check things out with others you trust.

Because each person is unique, be aware of your triggers and talk to your partner directly about them. Don't second-guess yourself and don't assume anything. This is a time to remember key aspects of the Four Cornerstones of Intimacy and put them into play. Remember to take a stand for what's true for you, comfort your anxieties, don't react to your partner's feelings, be assertive, speak up for yourself, and use empathy.

Old Patterns and a New Story

Many sex addicts learned through the neglect or trauma they experienced in their families of origin to get their needs met by being seductive and manipulative in relationships with others. Relating to people with sexual energy gave them a false sense of power and control. Since an addict's currency is sexuality, their motives are to control the outcome of a situation for self-gratification, whether it's with a boss, someone behind a checkout counter, or a lover.

As a recovering person, you've learned additional ways to relate to people, plus you've had the opportunity to make friends of the same gender through 12-step meetings. In these meetings, men tell me they much "prefer women because they understand me better." Women say they "prefer men because they're not catty, and I can trust them more." It's possible that both of these statements can be about running old patterns and manipulating the opposite sex in order to feel safe. Avoiding having same-sex friends can be a trap for people in recovery and a way to avoid dealing with intimacy issues, as demonstrated in Marie's story.

Marie had a competitive relationship with her mother growing up and into her addictive years as an adult. She traveled through life with a gaggle of ex-lovers whom she called friends. The truth was that Marie knew exactly how to seduce and manipulate these men into getting what she wanted and needed. This kept Marie in control of her "friendships." Learning to trust women, ask them for nurturing, and rely on them for her recovery was difficult but ultimately healing for Marie.

If you have friendships *only* with the opposite sex or past sexual partners, it's time to rethink your friendships. If you still don't have same-sex friends, ask yourself what stops you from doing so. This is an issue that is normally addressed in the early stages of recovery.

Conversely, a big step toward intimacy is making friends (of the opposite gender if you're heterosexual or the same gender if you're gay or lesbian) without sexualizing them or having sex with them. Have open and honest conversations about how you feel and what you enjoy about their company. They will help you become more assertive and authentic.

If you do sexualize someone you want to create a friendship with, acknowledge the feeling behind it and explore it more deeply. Ask yourself, "Where is my emotional pain, fear, or anger?" Pay attention to which stressors may be affecting you or the relationship.

Listen to how your friends respond, even though they may say things you don't want to hear. Realize that having explicit conversations about the boundaries and expectations of both parties is vital to your friendships' success.

Martin and Roxanne's Story

Early in their friendship, Martin told his new friend Roxanne that he just wanted to be friends. He was clear with himself that he did not find her attractive as a girlfriend. Also, he realized that certain fundamental behaviors wouldn't work for him in a long-term relationship. Martin also revealed his sexual recovery to her.

Roxanne said she had no difficulty with his sexual recovery, and she was attracted to him. When Martin insisted he wanted to stay platonic, she agreed. However, he didn't really listen to Roxanne's feelings. For six months they enjoyed each other's company, going to movies and riding bikes, yet Roxanne secretly hoped for more.

Over time, Martin lapsed into his patterns of seductive behaviors. Giving Roxanne signals such as hugs and affectionate touching, he was covertly tripping the sexual "green light." She read his signals as a go-ahead to become sexual. She thought that if they had sex, Martin would change his mind and desire a relationship with her. By passively allowing sex to happen with Roxanne, Martin had a major boundary failure. He lost his sobriety, ruined his friendship, and had to address his fears and discomfort about intimacy without sexualizing the relationship.

Have a Variety of Friends

As mentioned in Chapter 5, having a variety of sobriety-minded friends provides the opportunity for significant healing. For example, Jack, a former professional football player, joined a weekend men's football team. He loved playing but never felt comfortable hanging out with the guys afterward, so he'd simply disappear after a game. One Saturday, his teammates pressured him to join them at the local sports bar for a bite to eat. Jack bit the bullet and went with them. Afterward, he couldn't believe how much fun he'd had. "I didn't realize how important it was to hang out and shoot the breeze with the guys. It was liberating."

Similarly, don't be afraid to expect mutuality from friends. It's even okay to get into arguments if you're unhappy or have a misunderstanding. Stand up for yourself and learn to have the experience of repairing misunderstandings in safe and constructive ways. Above all, stay out of isolation. Otherwise, who would be there for you?

Rachel always had a difficult time confronting people and didn't trust anyone to be there for her. Like most sex addicts, she learned early on that she had to take care of her own needs. She was used to "stealing" her emotional needs by being passive-aggressive, meaning she would ignore the person who had affected her and then sneak around to get what she needed. When her friend Jenny told Rachel she couldn't help her paint her apartment over the weekend like she'd promised, Rachel got angry but told Jenny it was "fine." Instead of telling Jenny how disappointed and angry she was that Jenny didn't keep her commitment, Rachel chose to stop talking to Jenny by ignoring her phone calls.

In recovery, Rachel became tongue-tied when she had to tell others she wasn't happy about how they behaved toward her. Likewise, being direct about saying "thank you" was difficult when she received compliments. Why? Because Rachel was afraid if she told the truth, people wouldn't like her. She came to understand that she was afraid of telling Jenny how angry she was because she worried it would end the friendship. But freezing Jenny out by not talking to her almost *did* end the friendship.

Rachel learned she would have to make a point of speaking up in the moment, even though she might not get what she wanted or others might feel hurt or offended. At times, speaking her truth did upset her friends, but applying the Four Cornerstones of Intimacy allowed her to take a differentiated stand. Together, they could repair the rupture. Other times, Rachel found that when she was truthful, she received what she wanted. In addition, opening her heart to accept compliments by simply saying "thank you" began her journey toward self-valuation and seeing herself as more than a sex object.

Form Your Recovery Dating Plan

If you're single, now is the time to formulate a dating plan that can quell your fears and give you a positive focus. Many sex addicts in recovery skip important aspects of choosing and dating partners. Ignoring the process of deliberately choosing a partner undermines the potential for a healthy romantic relationship. Alternatively, a sound Recovery Dating Plan can clearly define a suitable or unsuitable partner and an appropriate timeline for healthy dating behavior. After you've gathered information about the person you are interested in, share it with your sponsor, friends, therapist, and other accountability partners. The following Recovery Dating Plan gives you a guide and a great place to start.

Part One: You

As you start, writing down your answers will help you become clear about what to look for when you're on a date. Consider your behaviors, warning signs, and deal breakers. Take this time to observe yourself as a person in recovery and be sure to live in your integrity.

In the grid below are three columns, Green, Yellow, and Red, which mean the following:

- **Green** represents your healthy behaviors.
- **Yellow** represents warning signs that you're being triggered in old ways or in your middle-circle behaviors, noted earlier. Your middle-circle behaviors are people, places, things, situations, or states of being that are hazardous to your recovery. These behaviors don't add to your recovery and can often prompt you to think about acting out.
- **Red** represents your deal breakers, or indicators that you're probably acting out.

Table 6.1. Recovery Dating Plan

Green (Healthy behaviors)	Yellow (Warning signs)	Red (Deal breakers)
• I genuinely look forward to seeing the person. • I tell the truth. • I take an active interest and ask questions to get to know the partner. • I compliment from a solid place in myself, not out of need. • I say "good night" in an appropriate way that feels good for me.	• I overspend to impress my date. • I obsess about what was said and examine every nuance. • I find myself trying to "fix" the other person or his/her problems. • I value the other's opinion or time more than my own. • I fantasize about our future together. • I rationalize not getting my needs met.	• I miss work or meetings to be with the person. • I lie about myself. • I lie by omission. • I become more isolated and my social circle is diminishing. • I rationalize a lot of middle-circle activity. • I find I'm not that interested in the person but go out anyway because I don't have any other prospects. • I have sex because I haven't had it in a long time.

Make a similar grid for yourself on a separate piece of paper. You'll find that the more items that fill out each column, the more useful your plan will be. Be rigorously honest in answering the question, "Is this person a healthy choice for me?" Be specific, as well as general, with your list.

Consider these questions:

- Are you adhering to your values and integrity?
- Are you being considerate?
- Are you acting out any of your addictive patterns of the past (such as trying to impress by overpaying or paying all the time)? If so, identify these behaviors and stop them.
- Do you want to immediately tell all about your addiction in order to manage your anxiety?
- Are you comforting your anxieties—or regressing emotionally?
- Is your sense of humor appropriate?
- Do you talk about interests and hobbies?

Part Two: The Partner

If you learn that the person you're currently dating is a recovering sex addict, I highly recommend setting boundaries and putting the Four Cornerstones of Intimacy into action before you proceed in the relationship. Then using the Recovery Dating Plan for Partners will assist you in taking a stand for what you need, comforting your anxieties, being assertive, and having emotional empathy.

In the grid for your plan are three columns: green is for ideal qualities, yellow for warning signs, and red for deal breakers. Again, make your own grid and fill in the columns regarding your dating partner. This exercise will guide your decision about proceeding in the relationship.

Be rigorously honest in answering the question, "What do I want in a partner?" Answer in detail as well as in general terms. Consider including the following: values/integrity, consideration for others, lifestyle, wreckage from past behaviors, possible addictions, education, emotional IQ, age range, sense of humor, interests/hobbies, relationships, spiritual beliefs, and family of origin. The more qualities you identify, the more useful your plan will be.

Table 6.2. Recovery Dating Plan for Partners

Green (Ideal qualities)	Yellow (Warning signs)	Red (Deal breakers)
• Is actively in recovery	• Doesn't return my calls in a timely manner	• Reports having unsafe sex
• Is on a path of self-awareness	• Is dating multiple people	• Devalues my program
• Is physically attractive to me	• Has a different faith when I know how important my own is	• Has a history of physical violence or gets violent in my presence
• Has similar interests		
• Is intellectually stimulating	• Doesn't have a job and hasn't held one for a while	• Steals from me
• Makes me laugh		• Is in relationship with someone else
• Shares my values about family, spirituality, etc.	• Appears aimless in his/her direction in life	• Has an active addiction
	• Seems chronically unhappy or complains a lot	• Constantly leaves me feeling bad about myself
		• Treats me poorly

Part Three: The Dating Timeline

Whether you're a sex addict in recovery or dating a sex addict in recovery, set a clear Dating Timeline to determine the right fit. Make a realistic plan for what your contact boundaries will be while dating. Again, be specific, as well as general, with your list and review it with your sponsor or another trusted friend in recovery.

With this Recovery Dating Plan, you're clear about who you are and what you want, making it easier to comfort your anxieties while on a date. Treat it as a blueprint to occasionally deviate from, not a plan set in stone. Use this as a resource to assist you in holding a differentiated stance, learning to trust your intuition, and maintaining recovery thinking.

Table 6.3. Dating Timeline

Dates 1–4 (1st month)	Dates 5–8 (2nd month)	Dates 19–15 (3rd month)
Talk on phone or e-mail 1–2 times a week max.	"Light" petting, above the waist (hands), outside clothes.	Discontinue dating others before having intercourse discussion.
No text messages.	French-kissing, being physically affectionate.	Disclose sexual history and addiction (before intercourse!).
Date others.		
Postpone serious talk about your history or past relationships.	Talk on phone or e-mail no more than 4–5 times a week.	Discuss STDs, HIV status, and birth control.
Hug, kiss on cheek.	Text messages used sparingly.	Have oral sex, intercourse (use condom).
Both take cars and meet there.	Seeing each other's house/home.	Sleep over at each other's house.
Share expenses or spend no more than $50–100 on a date.	Spend more than $100 on a date.	Short vacations (i.e., weekends away).

Jerry's Story

Jerry started dating in fits and starts at age thirty-seven after his recovery period. Feeling good about his sobriety and ready to commit to someone for the first time in his life, he "attacked" dating as if it were a contact sport. Still, he committed to others in his support group that he would follow the rules of his dating plan and timeline. He wanted to do this with integrity and meet Ms. Right.

Yet being the intensity seeker he was, he had difficulty settling himself down. In reality, his anxieties were running the show. He had a solid Recovery Dating Plan, but he kept deviating from it, trying avenues that weren't right for him. For example, his first date was a blind date, which was anxiety-provoking for him. The woman was attractive enough, but the evening fell apart quickly. Jerry felt no chemistry with her and didn't ask her out again. (In general, blind dates can be risky because you don't know whether or how you might be triggered by the other person. It's prudent to stay away from them in favor of meeting the person in a group through the people who want to set you up. When you're out in a group, there's less pressure to perform and you can converse with others if you feel no attraction toward the individual.)

He found his next date via the Internet. This woman was in recovery herself and talked nonstop about her drug addiction and the struggles she was having. Jerry got triggered! He recognized in her his pattern to rescue and ultimately act out with such a woman.

Finally, Jerry's support group encouraged him to slow down. Members of his group suggested that he tell everyone he knew that he was available and looking to date. They suggested he get together with prospective dates with friends present. Jerry agreed—no more blind dates or electronic dates for him. Deciding to go on dates with others present created a social life for Jerry outside of the recovery community, and he made new friends of both sexes.

Three months into the process, Jerry met a woman he enjoyed. Unsure about his physical attraction, he was still willing to get to know her on many levels. Because Sara was the sister of a friend, Jerry felt accountable for his behavior and made no move lightly.

On their first date—a midweek luncheon—Jerry discovered they had much in common, including shared values. Sara made him laugh in a way he hadn't laughed with anyone else. For the first month, Jerry experienced what it was like to actually court someone. He allowed himself to notice all the *firsts*—like the first time they held hands and kissed. He noted the laughter they shared and enjoyed Sara's sharp wit.

Jerry happily anticipated their time together and noticed his growing sexual attraction. As they grew closer, he saw old patterns of wanting to withdraw and run. That indicated his nervous system had to learn to tolerate intimacy and closeness when he tended to pull away. The group encouraged him to lean into the relationship and the good feelings he experienced, which seemed foreign and uncomfortable to him. Every time he got cold feet, he talked to Sara about his fears first. Jerry found himself slowly, magically falling in love with Sara.

Before long, Sara and Jerry were talking about their mutual attraction to each other, their desire to be boyfriend and girlfriend, and what that meant to each of them. They also talked about exclusivity, birth control, STDs, and, eventually, Jerry's sex addiction. Sara was curious and frightened about what this meant as it affected their coupleship. She wanted time to learn more about sex addiction and consider whether she wanted a relationship with him.

Frightened by her reaction, he feared he would lose her. He gave her the space she needed while admitting that in the past, he would have manipulated her into staying with him. This became an exercise in following the Four Cornerstones of Intimacy. In his desire to be a differentiated adult, he stood his ground like a champ and felt more self-respect than he could ever remember having before. He had been through enough recovery to know that chasing after her or groveling would make him feel chaotic and ashamed, which could lead to his acting out.

Sara needed time to talk to her closest friends, to be quiet within, and to review her own desires. She weighed the pros and cons, had several phone conversations with Jerry, in which he answered her questions, and decided to move ahead with the relationship.

Jerry decided to move forward with Sara, consulting his sponsor, group members, and friends every step of the way. When he became scared, he reached out. When he got anxious or fantasized that the grass was greener elsewhere or wanted to run, he reached out again. He worked hard to stay in the relationship by taking to heart the adage of "contrary action," that is, doing the opposite of one's first reaction. In this case, whenever Jerry had a reaction to run away from the relationship, he moved *toward* it.

Bill and Kristy's Story

Practicing the art of conversation is essential for achieving intimacy. Bill and Kristy, in their midforties, had first come together twenty years before when they were both drinking and using drugs. In fact, all their sexual encounters had been sex with substances. When they married, Kristy believed that both of them had stopped their drinking and drug usage.

Although Bill stopped drinking, he continued using drugs and started having sex with women he picked up in bars. In the meantime, Kristy became a stay-at-home soccer mom with three sons and one daughter. When she discovered Bill was having sex with strangers on his business trips and on invented fishing trips with his buddies, the relationship blew apart.

The couple went through the whole recovery process and they endeavored to have sex again. Kristy felt uncomfortable with her body because the only *erotic* sex she'd ever known with Bill was drunken sex. Kristy remembered sex being "hot" between the two of them when they were drunk. This was her only experience of sex that felt free and where she felt a sense of abandon. The sex they'd had over the years since their marriage was described by them as "fairly ordinary," since neither one of them had been emotionally present. Over time, they'd found excuses to have sex less often. In recovery, Kristy had to deal with her shame and discomfort, which came from early childhood traumas and inappropriate sexual messages from her family.

In some ways, Bill's absence from the marriage kept Kristy from ever having to face her sexuality as an adult woman. She could focus on raising her kids and complain about Bill's neglect of her because he was never home, ostensibly because of his busy career. In no way was it Kristy's fault that Bill acted out sexually, but in many ways it colluded with her denial around her discomfort with her sexuality. Their recovery task revolved around lots of conversations like these: "What are we doing now? We've already had kids. We committed to stay in the marriage. However, our kids are growing and headed away from home. I'm grappling with the question of whether I really want to stay or leave. I'm asking myself, *Why do I want to stay? Why would I stay? What are we here to do with each other?*"

Bill and Kristy's choices might involve recommitment—or perhaps commitment for the first time, because they hadn't been in an honest marriage from day one. Let's look at the process they went through to discover what they wanted.

When you recommit to your partner, start dating, or seek a relationship, you'll rely on your values, which generally remain the same throughout life, even as your circumstances change. Your agreements should be congruent with your values. If you're dating, you'll have to decide what values you firmly believe in to guide your choices and actions. Look again at how you trampled on those values in your addiction and decide how you will rewrite your story.

In the addiction period, you were incongruent with your values, but that's part of the addict's shame. In Bill's case, he put his family life, career, and wife and children in jeopardy through his actions. When your values are congruent with your actions, you no longer say one thing and do another. This is key for rebuilding trust in your relationship. Your actions must match your words. When you have integrated the disparate parts of your personality, you become whole.

Perhaps the rigid values you held while in your active addictions were based on what you thought you were supposed to do and be, according to your family of origin. As a sober person, you get to reevaluate—to create a new value system that's specific to who you are, what you believe, and what you want.

From all viewpoints, Bill was a successful businessman. Others saw him and Kristy as a happy couple. However, his addictive behavior was the myopic vision of a hijacked brain, which creates a gigantic blind spot in the addict's perception. Thinking in a sober way had Bill saying, "I can't believe I actually damaged myself and my family the way I did. I don't ever want to do that again." With that intention and clear thought, Bill can reexamine his values and use them to guide the next cycle of intimacy with Kristy.

What's happening? In addiction, the brain function controlling good moral decision making has gone "off line." That means little blood and oxygen flow to that part of the brain because the brain's reward center is getting the lion's share, thus usurping good values and good judgment. In this case, Bill's values might have been solidly in place while he was acting out sexually, but his addiction had the upper hand.

In recovery, while individual values may remain the same, you must reconvene, converse, and make a recommitment to coupleship. Take time to discuss with each other what your values mean. In Bill's case, he needs to rethink his values and talk to Kristy about them. Although he believed his values before recovery were worthy, he couldn't uphold them. For example, Bill grew up believing that "honesty was the best policy," yet in his addiction, he sometimes lied to coworkers and friends, and lied all the time to his wife concerning his whereabouts. He couldn't uphold the value of honesty. In recovery, he decided that the value of honesty was crucial to his integrity, so he chose to live daily as an honest man—no secrets, no lies.

On the other hand, his value of perfectionism created problems for him. Bill decided that being rigid was not healthy. He gave himself breathing room to live his life honestly but imperfectly. In his addiction, Bill often made excuses for why he had to come home late and used that time to act out. As part of his commitment to honesty and accountability, he chose to call Kristy when he left the office every night at the same time to let her know when he would be home. On occasion, he would get distracted by a phone call and forget to call her. In early recovery, Kristy got upset and angry, but over time she learned to calm down. These days, she waits fifteen minutes before she starts calling him. Bill doesn't beat himself up if he forgets to call, allowing for the imperfection of his humanity.

What values do you think couples renegotiate when they're in recovery and moving on? Which of your values are up for reconsideration? Consider the following discussion about values as you answer these questions for yourself.

The Value of Values

Sexuality changes within a relationship, so you cannot presume to know a lot about it. When starting your conversations, it's best to come together with a clear mind. Remember, you probably know very little about your own sexuality because it was arrested at an early age, and you may have been repeating the same rigid patterns for years.

Because sexuality changes, coming together for intimate sexual pleasuring means to remain open and be present with your partner. Paradoxically, your personal values remain stable because you are congruent in your life choices. *This means you are who you say you are and you do what you say you will do.*

Another paradox is that when you experiment sexually, you may bump up against values that no longer serve you because they've become too restrictive for your expanding growth. Those values may have kept you from taking risks and growing into an adult sexually; now they limit you.

For example, sex addicts can hold the value that their wives should maintain a certain kind of modesty that doesn't allow for sexual experimentation. This value can collude with the addicts' fears and shame, giving them an excuse to have sex outside of the relationship. Remembering the Four Cornerstones of Intimacy: self-knowledge, comfort and connection, responsibility with discernment, and empathy with emotion help in a number of ways. You can accept what you like sexually without judgment, tell your partner about it without reacting to his or her response, and have empathy for your partner's feelings. By being honest, you can begin to set new values that are congruent with who you want to be sexually and the kind of sexual partner you would like to be. This level of honesty puts you on the road to a hot, healthy sex life.

Following is a chart that will help you define your values and visions both as an individual and as a couple. If you are single, I recommend you follow Step 1 by choosing ten values, then follow Step 2 and prioritize your top six values. Consider doing this exercise with a close friend and share your lists with one another. This will assist you in getting clear about your values for your future relationship.

Here's what to do:

1. As a couple, claim up to ten of the values listed that define your viewpoint or that you believe in strongly.
2. Then, as an individual, prioritize your top six values from the list of ten you make together in their order of importance to you.

3. Next, share your lists with each other and notice if any of the values you've chosen overlap. Combine your lists into a Coupleship Values List, which doesn't have to be in any particular order. Try to keep your combined list to at least five but no more than seven values. Work together so you hear each other, and be clear about what is nonnegotiable for you and what you can let go.

4. Finally, repeat the steps above to create a second combined list that will comprise your Sexual Values List, which will serve to guide your sex life.

Table 6.4. Values and Visions Chart

Integrity	Mastery	Play	Joy	Authenticity
Adventure	Loyalty	Education	Leadership	Nurturance
Cleanliness	Collaboration	Self-care	Creativity	Discipline
Beauty	Resilience	Directness	Privacy	Compassion
Determination	Romance	Free Spirit	Spirituality	Health
Intimacy	Success	Honesty	Service	Humor
Vitality	Trust	Tradition	Well-being	Learning
Productivity	Happiness	Intelligence	Religion	Freedom to Choose

Susan and Charlie's Story

Susan and Charlie are artists with solid careers. They value beauty and aesthetics but also have a strong work ethic. Together they made their value list and then prioritized their separate lists of six. Susan's list included loyalty, honesty, spirituality, intimacy, aesthetics, and humor. Charlie had productivity at the top of his list, along with aesthetics, adventure, honesty, and learning.

When they merged their lists of values, they decided that loyalty, honesty, aesthetics, spirituality, productivity, and humor would guide their coupleship. Susan and Charlie found several cooperative ways to ritualize those qualities in their daily lives. They decided to meditate together every morning and every night, and they agreed to tell each other one thing they did that day, thus illustrating their loyalty to each other. As a way to exemplify honesty, Charlie chose to check in with Susan on a regular basis and tell her of his whereabouts and who was with him. Feeling grateful that laughter had returned to their marriage, they made efforts to make each other laugh.

They chose intimacy, adventure, freedom to choose, aesthetics, and learning to guide their sex life. They applied these values to their sex life by talking about how they could practice each value while being sexual, and what each one meant to them.

Your assignment is to do as Susan and Charlie did—create your own joint values chart and discuss the values in it. Answer these three questions, add your answers to your stories, and bring the answers to your conversations with your partner.

- Which values would you like to adopt to guide your coupleship?
- Which values could relate to your sex life?
- How do you both define your values, and how will you put them into practice?

✓ Erotic Intelligence Checklist for Chapter 6

❑ Learn to nurture opposite-gender friends without sexualizing or having sex with them. This is a big step toward intimacy. Have open and honest conversations with your friends about how you feel and what you enjoy about their company.

❑ Plan important aspects of returning to dating after recovery. A sound Recovery Dating Plan includes: (1) determining healthy and unhealthy behaviors, (2) defining characteristics and behaviors of suitable and unsuitable partners, and (3) planning an appropriate timeline for healthy dating behavior.

❑ Reevaluate or create a value system that's specific to who you are, what you believe, and what you want. Both as an individual and as a couple, determine your main values. Then talk about how your mutual values can be expressed in your coupleship and in your sex life together.

CHAPTER

7

Integrating
Love and Healthy Lust

Lust is desire for the body;
love is desire for the soul.

—Author Unknown

In Chapter 6 you took initial steps to start conversations about your values, vision, priorities, and expectations for your relationship as a couple. Now it's time to move toward an integration of love and lust in healthy, intimate ways. Understanding the difference between the two will help you create a picture of your journey ahead.

Cultural Sexual Messages

The 1970s brought us "wife swapping" or "swinging" in the midst of people raising families. Kids were left to "do their own thing," while adults kept trying to "find themselves." Women juggled careers and families—and sometimes affairs. The 1980s loosened attitudes even more. Competition became the name of the corporate game. Cocaine use was overtly fashionable, and the accumulation of material wealth hit new heights.

All this "openness" brought a new level of promiscuity, accompanied by HIV and AIDS. While millions of people died of this dreaded disease, others continued to dance, drink, and snort cocaine into the wee hours of the decade. By the 1990s, the modern women's battle cry was, "You can have it all: marriage, children, career, and sexual freedom!"

Today, we preach abstinence to our youth in sex education, yet our culture has become more sexualized because we're bombarded with "adult" images. On the one hand, we get the message that sex should be reserved for the one we love, while on the other, advertisements, movies, and billboards encourage us to sexualize ourselves. This paradox pulls people in two directions. They report feeling tired and burned out. They say they don't have time to spend with their families and can't maintain a healthy lifestyle. They turn to other sexual outlets as a form of escape.

The highly sexualized parts of our culture have given everyone access to the erotic and the pornographic: films at the press of a button on the remote, billboards advertising "Gentlemen's Clubs," phone sex, and prostitutes-to-order. We can meet and have sex with strangers; we can even interact sexually with people via webcams on our computers.

Sexual Messages Abound

Sex addicts aren't created in a vacuum. The unending sexual messages we get from film, TV programs, magazines, billboards, fashion, and the Internet—plus issues related to trauma from our families—create a recipe for the making of a sex addict. These factors have made sex addiction a prolific and painful problem, both socially and personally. In fact, sexual addiction (specifically pornography addiction) has been referred to by Dr. Patrick Carnes as our newest and most challenging mental health problem.

The media advocate upholding family values while also hawking goods and services to keep us perennially young. Being sexy and holding on to youth have become integral to the consumer culture and contribute to the economy. The result? We're left feeling *less than* after being hypnotized with the more-is-better message: more money, more sexiness, more success, more corrective surgeries to achieve that sexiness. With this relentless bombardment, the reward system of our brain is constantly signaling "novelty." With each release of dopamine, excitement is created that has us wanting even more. It seems that our collective reward system has gone haywire.

For many, *more* is simply not enough.

Chronic Novelty Seekers

By now, you know that sex addicts endlessly seek novelty. You've experienced the hijacked brain. When the reward system that produces dopamine is constantly engaged, as it is with novelty, you feel the intensity that's the hallmark of sex addiction. Over time, however, this sort of novelty seeking creates despondence, a kind of dangerous exhaustion, or an uncomfortable mania.[1]

The Internet, an extraordinary invention that allows us to learn, grow, and connect with people all over the world, also provides sex at our fingertips. Sexual images and engagement are available in our homes and offices with the click of a mouse. But cybersex can deeply affect our brains and sexual actions. Virtual connections without face-to-face contact allow for sexual exchanges to happen in our imagination and devoid of any heart connection. This reinforces addictive patterns and the lack of real relationship interactions. Forming attachments to pixel screens and fantasy avatars leaves novelty seekers feeling isolated, lonely, and unsatisfied.

In *The Porn Trap*, authors Wendy and Larry Maltz write, "Powerful human bonding hormones, such as oxytocin and vasopressin, are released with orgasm. They contribute to establishing a lasting emotional attachment with whomever or *whatever* you happen to be with or you're thinking about at the time. The more orgasms you have with porn, the more sexually and emotionally attached to it you'll become."[2]

People in sexual recovery have had to show tremendous fortitude in their environments. Initially, they must constantly fight against the tendencies to medicate their pain; plus, they must face the shock of discovery by their partner or the shock of admitting to themselves that they are hurting. However, no matter how difficult it may be to navigate the pressures of society and the painful realizations of recovery, the power of choice can overcome them.

Yet what remains true is this: *You can develop your unique story, make fresh choices, and experience the sexual intimacy you desire.* You simply have to learn how. Chapters 10 and 11 will open up new levels of intimacy to you.

Rebuilding Your Relationship

Having pledged to a life of integrity, you're now committing to the spirit of coupleship. You've taken the high road to recovery. Moving nobly into the growth phase of your relationship has you walking with your dignity intact, perhaps for the first time in your life.

To walk together *as a couple* with your heads held high can pose yet another challenge. Many partners of addicts have told me they feel bad about themselves for staying in the relationship because of the betrayal they've experienced. They imagine that the people who know their past judge them to be stupid for staying with the person who's caused them so much pain. I often counter this thinking, explaining that leaving may seem quick and easy because they can pretend they're okay and the problem has disappeared. However, if you leave your relationship, you'll be stuck with your pain and sorrow *without* the person you loved to help you sort it out. Why is this true? Because even though it feels as if your pain comes from your partner, it's actually coming from inside you.

Staying is another story altogether. You have to walk in the unknown with no guarantees. You're asked daily to show up for your life and see what's there, not to make any swift moves. You tread lightly and trust the process with awareness. With each passing day, you experience a glimmer of a new beginning in yourself and in the other person. You begin to have a relationship with yourself as a whole being and wisely recognize yourself as the source of your happiness.

However, if you don't see changes in your partner, or your partner is treating you poorly, then it's time to consider leaving. At this juncture, you should have serious conversations with your trusted friends, sponsor, and therapist. While difficult and painful, leaving may be the best decision for your personal growth and development.

Sexual Potential in Coupleship

You're no longer having sex as a compulsive need to feel good, and your sex life may be functional. But how do you go beyond just "functional" to experience sexual fulfillment? Let's examine what Doug and Samantha have done to improve intimacy.

Doug and Samantha's Story

Doug and Samantha had been married for fifteen years when Samantha uncovered Doug's numerous affairs. In their forties, with two adolescent boys, as a couple they struggled with their sexuality. Doug moved out of the house for a year while they worked on their relationship in hopes of keeping their marriage and family intact.

Although she felt furious and hurt, Samantha loved Doug and wanted to make things work. Plagued by her own eating disorder, she struggled with not overreacting and medicating her feelings with food. Her own body image stood in the way of her desire to be sexual with Doug. In addition, she had many underlying family-of-origin issues to face.

Doug's tendency was to intimidate and cajole Samantha into getting what he wanted sexually. He knew his patterns and believed he had successfully changed them.

One night after Doug had moved back home, he and Samantha decided to have sex. They both felt awkward and uncomfortable being sexual with each other but didn't talk about their discomfort. Instead, they rushed into having sex with little eye contact and no kissing or heart connection.

During the sex act, Doug's dissociation caused him to revert to old patterns of objectification with no connection, telling Samantha he was going to "lick your pussy." Livid, Samantha felt used, but she continued in the sexual act. Afterward, they told each other that they had experienced orgasms, but they both felt terrible. He admitted feeling disconnected and empty, while Samantha confessed to feeling alone and violated. Doug realized he had reverted to old patterns and that he couldn't say phrases like "lick your pussy" to her when he had no emotional connection with her. From her side, she felt terribly unloved but chose to attempt having sex anyway, which went against being true to herself. In fact, neither one of them took responsibility for themselves from the initial point of awkwardness onward.

Using the Four Cornerstones of Intimacy, self-knowledge, comfort and connection, responsibility with discernment, and empathy with emotion, in therapy, they isolated this bad experience to learn about themselves and move toward their sexual potential as a couple. Uncomfortable as intimate conversations were for them, they understood that they had to talk about their fears and anxieties as a way to build intimacy *before* becoming sexual with each other.

Exploring sexual potential means having deep conversations about what is possible. Remember, in your addiction, you constantly pursued achieving the ultimate orgasm. In so doing, you missed the possibility of eroticism, which is transcendent and intimate, leading you closer to yourself, your partner, and the divine.

In sexual sobriety, you create your new story by constantly striving for ideal goals. You're disciplined because you define certain practices that you follow daily and weekly.

Together, you and your partner will define your values, personal intentions, and goals as a couple and start a journey to fulfill them. You accept that intercourse is not the be-all and end-all. Rather, seeing each other in true "nakedness" and being willing to share your fears and desires leads to the joy of sexual fulfillment.

Vision Statement for Coupleship Intimacy

Couples who create a vision statement for coupleship bring their hearts and ideas together for one purpose—sexual intimacy. Their vision statement helps them evaluate if they're successfully moving toward the vision they have for their life together. They create and use their vision statement as a guide for many goals in life. Using this statement of intention, each partner can be accountable to his or her own commitments. This accountability can serve as a comfort as well as a challenge and is well worth pursuing.

If you are single, a vision statement is especially useful as you prepare to get involved in a sexual relationship. Clearly setting your vision for the kind of person and relationship you would like to attract will assist you in giving yourself permission to be sexual and seek healthy sexual relations when the time is right.

Creating Your Vision Statement

Take the values you've distilled from Chapter 6 and incorporate them into your vision statement. It can be any length that feels right for you—a sentence, a paragraph, even several pages. Write a statement that includes your values and goals for yourself and your coupleship using the guidelines below. Remember, your values and goals may shift over time as you grow as individuals and together as a couple. For now, craft your vision according to what you're thinking and feeling today. Make your statement(s) practical and fun for both of you.

- "Where do we want to end up together?" (Examples: growing old together; traveling around the world together; continuing our spiritual realization as a couple.)
- "How do I want to see myself?" (Examples: I wish to see myself as a grandfather, happily married, and enjoying retirement; I see myself as returning to school for my degree and opening my own business, coming home to my supportive, sexy husband; I see myself continuing to desire my sexy wife and having an enriching, meaningful life with her while pursuing my dream of learning to sail.)
- How would you like your partner to see you and what might he or she say about you in five or ten years? (Examples: She looks great to me; I find him as sexy and desirable as ever; she's my friend and a true companion whom I can count on.)
- Place your emphasis on what has the most meaning to you and what you can reasonably do.
- State what you intend not to do again as a reminder. (Examples: I choose to never again lie or cheat on my partner; I choose to never again forget to tell her I love her on a daily basis; I choose to never again call him names that are destructive to him, my dignity, or our relationship.)
- What strengths do you bring to intimacy in coupleship? List several in priority order.

- What weaknesses do you need to work on? List several in priority order.
- What are your shared goals for connection? Do they include expressing affection, such as touching and active listening?

In addition, write down specific shared goals for spending time together. How much time in a week, month, and year can you commit to? Can you commit to taking one day each week as exclusively yours, perhaps calling it a date night?

Build Sexual Agreements into Your Vision Statement

Now that you've completed your vision statement for yourself and your coupleship, incorporate your own sexual vision statement. Use the values you chose from Chapter 6 along with this guide to create agreements you would like to have.

If you are single, think about these sexual agreements as sexual boundaries you might consider when entering a relationship. Talk to others who have begun dating or have gotten married while in recovery. Ask them to share what their sexual boundaries and needs were and how they communicated them.

As you do this, consider these examples of agreements couples have used in their sexual vision statement:

- Sex has to feel honest to both partners and aim to increase intimacy.
- No sexual activity outside of the committed relationship.
- No secrets or lies about sex, sexuality, or sexual preferences.

- Agree to be free to choose when and where they have sex.
- Agree to name their sexual limitations and work on areas where each partner feels stuck.
- Agree on why they have sex (e.g., to connect with each other; for pleasure, exploration, and discovery; to celebrate their love; to enjoy a sense of play, and so on).
- Agree to be clear on the different kinds of sex they want to have and what they don't want to have (e.g., take an afternoon or evening to slowly explore and build their sexual repertoire; have "maintenance sex," meaning sex that is more like what they usually enjoy, keeping connection in mind; have the occasional "quickie," meaning sex for the sake of quick pleasure, again with connection between the two of them).
- Agree to be present and allow for whatever happens without judgment.

You agree to your chosen values about your sexuality so that trust can serve as the foundation for trying new sexual behaviors. These new behaviors can lead to nervous tension when the opportunity for sex arises, so remember the third cornerstone of intimacy; comfort and connection. It will help you continue to develop the capacity to comfort your anxieties and connect with your partner without reacting to his or her feelings. It also allows you to love deeply while admitting to and experiencing the lust you feel for each other.

Integrating Healthy Lust and Love

When you are secure in yourself, know what turns you on, and enjoy watching your partner watch you experience sexual pleasure, you have a highly novel relationship grounded in love. The experience of seeing and being seen fuels lust and desire. This is exactly the way you integrate healthy lust and love into your sex life. It's *relational* sex, not the old pornographic sex of past addictions.

Loving deeply by looking into each other's eyes for prolonged periods actually stimulates novelty in the brain and affects the nervous system, either calming or arousing it. Our brains and bodies are wired to read cues from one another. Face-to-face closeness with your lover signals safety to the brain, which will have a calming effect on both of you. It's part of the attachment process discussed in Chapter 1.

Likewise, the brain can recognize lustful intention. Seducing your partner with your eyes can activate your own arousal as the reward system scans, signals novelty, and releases dopamine. Your partner receives your seductive signals, his/her brain/body responds, then your brain/body receives your partner's signal. This becomes a feedback loop. You're releasing dopamine and other sex hormones that create sexual arousal in the body. You're dancing the dance of intimacy and eroticism to the music of real connection.

Recognize Your Partner as a Sexual Being

When they're in their addiction, sex addicts constantly objectify and sexualize people. They report looking at "bodies," not people as individuals. They might watch a woman fill her gas tank at the self-serve pump or check out a guy cycling down the street and then go home and masturbate to that image. Sex addicts often hoard images of people for later use.

I encourage recovering addicts to think about how sexualizing and objectifying people can trigger them to act out. In early recovery, you were probably introduced to a strategy called the "three-second rule." As mentioned earlier, it allows you to have three seconds to notice how attractive a person is and then look away. Notice and look away. No gawking and going into fantasy. Instead, you learn to use the three-second rule as a cognitive intervention. This is how you'd work it: "In the first second, I acknowledge an attractive person. In the following second, I admit I'm a sex addict and the other person's body is none of my business. In the third second, I pray for the other person's health and happiness. I also remind myself that person didn't give me permission to sexualize his/her body."

Another action strategy is to see your partner as the beautiful, powerful sexual being that he or she is. Remember, sex is no longer driven by your secret fantasy or genital focus, but by what's happening between the two of you. *It's relational.* Talk to your partner about what it's like for you to regard him or her as a sexual being. Viewing yourself as a sexual being and allowing your partner to see you as such may require the second cornerstone of intimacy—that you comfort your anxieties so that you can grow sexually.

Be sure to sincerely compliment your partner before you sexualize him or her. You do this to emphasize you want *him* or *her*, not the person you just saw on the street. That way, sex becomes healthier as you bring to it a sense of play and joy. And to make it work, remember the small details. Notice and compliment your partner, and express your appreciation aloud on a regular basis.

On the other end, if you have trouble receiving compliments, ask yourself these questions and share your answers with your partner:

- Do you shy away and withdraw, feel shame, and rebuff your partner's advance?
- Do you want to make your partner out to be lewd or inappropriate because he's checking you out?
- Can you accept the compliment and respond in flirtatious ways?

• What does it feel like to be seen as a sexual being from the person you love? Can you revel and delight in that?

Implicit Versus Explicit Expression of Love

"When having lunch with your partner or seeing him pick up your child, do you notice his beautiful smile or expressive eyes? Do you catch a certain glimpse that reminds you why you really love him?" In therapy, when I ask this question of my clients, they often respond that they do catch such glimpses that spur their love. When I ask if they tell their partner, they typically say "no."

I encourage people in recovery to use the implicit-explicit strategy, which means to say what's on your mind in a clear and practical way—an absolute necessity in relationships. "Implicit" refers to holding your thoughts inside, which is appropriate if you're considering your chess moves or have to keep a poker face to win a game of cards. To make your thoughts "explicit" in relationships means to start critical conversations and stay present with the process.

The key to being explicit is speaking the way you do with people in the program. You risk telling others that you care about them, that you appreciate their help, or that you're upset with them. And you congratulate them when they reach benchmarks in their sobriety. Recovery teaches you that you deserve to feel good, proud, and valuable. Once you feel that internally, then you share it with others and gift them with your experience, strength, and hope.

Now it's time to extend your generosity to your partner. Let her know how beautiful she is; tell him how grateful you are for what he did today; announce how proud you are for both of your accomplishments. Don't be stingy. Sensuality desires and calls for a lavish abundance of words, thoughts, and feelings.

Raise the energy through a sense of play and by using the language of eroticism. Play with each other in loving, adoring, and respectful ways, but also raunchy ways. "Raunchy" means earthy, sexual, sensual, and explicit. Men are more likely to use raunchy language than women because it has an animalistic quality they find arousing. Remember, sexual language comes from the emotional centers of the brain and words can stimulate arousal. Usually, if women feel loved and respected, they won't be offended by raunchy language. If they are, they're wise to take the time to ask themselves why.

Intimacy Conversations Start with You

I suggest you start the intimacy conversation with yourself, then follow up with your partner. Intimate conversations with your partner move you into intimate sex, which can be playful, pleasurable, and deeply satisfying for both of you. This sort of intimacy rewards you with contentment and comfort; both of you feel safe within the love of your relationship. The next step, discussed in Chapter 8, is exploring erotic sex, bringing lust into love—a dynamic duo.

Typically, I hear men say, "I wish she was more wild and uninhibited" and women say, "I wish he was more relational." Don't despair. Both genders can look at any disowned part and start to change. The goal is to meet in the arena of eroticism, which is different from the arena of intimate love, but includes it. Being able to say to your wife, "You've got a great ass," or "I think you're hot," is important in the language of eroticism. But men and women recovering from sex addiction understand that until they can repair the heart and the love damaged by their disconnection, they won't talk in those ways or do those things.

If at any time the content of this material triggers you to want to replicate your sexually addictive behaviors—stop. Talk about it with your partner or someone in your program and work through what's going on with you. Ask yourself what makes you feel vulnerable and how these feelings keep you from changing or taking risks. Nothing should give you license to act out within the confines of your relationship.

Jill and Roger's Story

Unlike Doug and Samantha (from earlier in this chapter), Jill and Roger had several conversations about:

- Why they chose each other in the first place
- Why they were committing to each other again
- What would be different this time
- Their values and the purpose of their relationship
- Their vision for the future

Going through this process made them keenly aware of their differences, fears, and interests. Roger, an African American, was initially attracted to Jill, a Japanese American, because of her beauty and his fixation on Asian women, which she never knew. Although nervous to tell her, Roger admitted it was true. He explained how her slight frame and demure manner made him feel virile and masculine. Dominating her aroused him sexually.

Jill was able to hear his confession because she had become differentiated through her own recovery process. She better trusted herself, knew what was true for her, and saw Roger change over the past year. She also trusted that through their recovery, they had built a strong emotional and relational connection.

Jill admitted that she loved feeling protected by Roger and was aroused by his skin color and masculinity. They had never talked about these characteristics during their courtship, but had played them out implicitly in their marriage.

However, the problem was that Roger devalued Jill and lied to her while in his addiction. He didn't understand his attraction to her and felt shame for wanting dominant sex with her. His solution was to avoid sex with her altogether and visit Asian prostitutes, which made Jill feel powerless, unsafe, and unattractive.

When they could admit the truth to each other and build intimacy, they were able to bring all their desires into their sex life. Jill embraced her physical attributes and felt sexually alive again. She also knew he was extremely turned on by her, so she didn't hold back her sexuality. Roger, on the other hand, no longer felt shame about his attraction to Jill's body shape and size. He knew he honestly loved her and felt more entitled to his desire while knowing Jill wanted a future with him.

Repairing the Heart

Repairing your sex life after the ravages of sex addiction is not for the weak of heart. Therefore, what's your first task? *To repair your heart.* This is necessary, because partners often compare themselves to the people the sex addict acted out with. Addicts are often terrified to become sexually vulnerable, sometimes wanting to avoid sex altogether. But understand that the process of moving from healthy sex to intimate sex to erotic sex doesn't necessarily happen in perfect order. Sometimes one or both partners hit a wall when it comes to a deeper, more erotic exploration of their sexuality, as the case study with Sondra and James shows.

Sondra and James's Story

Keeping the Four Cornerstones of Intimacy in mind, Sondra and James dared to take on the challenges of their sex life and do it imperfectly. James, however, ran up against a wall. In the meantime, Sondra was bothered about the kind of sex they were having. Although she felt it was connected, loving, and functional, she missed the hot sex they'd enjoyed when they'd first met five years earlier. Besides, she didn't know that during their marriage, James had been hiring prostitutes on business trips as a matter of course.

Before learning about James's sex addiction, Sondra had been sexually adventurous and free. She didn't have sexual hang-ups about her body and loved giving and receiving pleasure. But finding out about James's sex addiction deeply affected her. She became enraged and left him, threatening divorce. This rocked James to his core, believing he'd lost the one thing that mattered most to him in the world—his marriage to Sondra. Three years into their recovery, they repaired their relationship, but it took a long time before James believed she wouldn't leave again.

Sondra finally recommitted to her marriage, but she felt inhibited and scared, concerned that their sex life would be boring. She wanted more aggressive, erotic sex, but didn't want to trigger James's acting out with another woman. She worried that she would never measure up to his ideas of "sexy" or be able to compete with the prostitutes.

In therapy, James listened to Sondra with an open mind and heart, being adultlike without collapsing into shame. He validated her desire to move into what Sondra called "X-rated sex" with him but said he wasn't quite ready to do that. James spoke truthfully when he confessed that the sex during his addiction was not glamorous, and he wouldn't return to it. He cherished the loving, connected sex they were having now and felt present with her.

Both acknowledged they were afraid to face their limitations. Sondra had to believe that she was sexy and desirable even though she wanted healthy approval from James. He had to risk stepping into uncomfortable arenas, trusting it wouldn't lead him to act out again.

The Brain: The Biggest Sex Organ

Men appear to be more sexually stimulated through visual means. Typically, males respond genitally to specific sexual stimuli that appeals to them. This usually means that sexual arousal is dependent on visuals that correspond to their sexual orientation and sexual preferences.[3]

For women, sexual arousal appears to be different than for men. Women are more likely to be genitally aroused by less specific sexual stimuli.[4] And when it comes to orgasm, Beverly Whipple, coauthor of *The Science of Orgasm*, researched how the brain produces orgasms and which biological processes are involved. Her book brings us up to date from what seems like the ancient definition of orgasm focused in the genitals. Today we know that orgasm for women can be clitoral, vaginal, or blended, and that orgasms without touch can happen through imagery and fantasy, verifying that orgasm happens mostly in the brain, not the body.

In addition, Whipple and her coauthors reviewed and validated the research concerning the location and purpose of the G-spot in women. They further concluded that pressure on the G-spot reduced pain during intercourse. Her groundbreaking work also revealed that women with spinal cord injuries can have orgasm.[5] Clearly, understanding genital arousal for men and women, and the process of orgasm for women, can help couples talk more knowledgeably and freely about how they both enjoy being stimulated, aroused, touched, and talked to.

If you haven't shared all of your sexual desires by now, take this time to stop and reveal yourself to your partner. What have you been afraid to share with him or her? Define those things and express them. Also express the erotic activities you'd like to engage in with your partner and have your partner do the same. Talk about them and prioritize doing them. You may be happily surprised to find that you share mutual desires. Sharing an open line of communication enhances your sexual relationship better than any other factor. Remember, sexually explicit conversation about what turns you on is a key to your intimacy in coupleship.

✓ Erotic Intelligence Checklist for Chapter 7

❏ Creating vision statements for yourself and with your partner for your coupleship and your shared sex life helps you evaluate whether or not you're successful in achieving your goals and keeping your commitments.

❏ Lust is a healthy response when two people feel loved, respected, and connected to each other.

❏ Understanding the physical and mental processes of arousal in both sexes can facilitate the all-important conversations that lead to greater fulfillment.

8

Pillow Talk
and Much More

Make love with the whole of yourself.
Bring your innocence and experience to the
bedroom. Be pure of heart and lust for your
lover. Hold out the promise of thrills—
and the comfort of safety, all at once.
Don't try, just do.

—Philip T. Sudo (1959–)

Pillow talk brings you to a deeper level of risking and exploring boundaries. Imagine you and your partner are awake in the early-morning hours before the busy day starts, or you're lying together in the late-night hours before slumber sets in. Your quiet privacy presents a good opportunity for pillow talk—straightforward, honest sharing and heartfelt discussions.

Congratulations on the work you've done thus far. It will help you navigate the tasks at hand without being triggered or reacting to your partner.

Say No Respectfully

While "pillow talk" can encompass any type of talk you have in bed, three aspects of pillow talk are essential to your well-being. The first is being able to say no, meaning it, and having your boundaries respected. The second includes saying yes, being heard, and following through. The third involves offering an alternate plan if the one that's being presented to you is not right in the moment. All three aspects are vital to maintaining a positive connection with yourself and your partner.[1]

Because shame has most likely had a stranglehold over your sexuality for a long time, responding to your partner in more authentic and vulnerable ways requires courage. Consider these suggestions:

- Listen with an open mind and heart: no blame, no shame. Be mindful of what it takes for your partner to stick his or her neck out and ask for what he or she needs.
- Take time to appreciate your partner's invitation to try a new technique that you may not be in the mood for.
- Never place judgment on the sexual act your partner requests. Saying things like "That's disgusting" or "It's immoral," or rolling your eyes doesn't help to diminish your fears, discomfort, and limitations regarding the sexual act. Projecting your judgments onto your partner only shames your partner and gets you off the hook of looking at yourself.
- It's always okay to say no, but be mindful about how you say it. For example, if your partner wants to have oral sex and you

don't, then decline with honesty and offer an alternate plan like, "I'm glad that idea turns you on, but I'm tired and want sex to be quick tonight. Can I take a rain check for the weekend?" Another response might be, "I understand that you're turned on by rear-entry vaginal sex, and I may want to try that with you later, but I'm not sure you're really connecting with me in that position. Until I feel more trusting of you, I want to wait."

Offer an alternate plan when it comes to touch as well. For example, if your partner is rubbing you in a way that feels good at first but begins to feel irritating, then communicate that you would like a lighter touch or prefer to be touched on another part of your body.

Mainly, talk to your partner about your personal experience and what you need to keep the sexual interaction open. If you're on the receiving end of the alternate plan, don't take it as rejection of you. Instead, hear the message as an invitation to comfort your anxieties while staying connected to your partner. It's also an opportunity to practice empathy for your partner's feelings and preferences.

These three keys to honest pillow talk leave both of you feeling heard and loved, not ignored and blamed:

1. *Use the language of "I" statements* to express your truth or feelings without judgment. For example, you might say, "I'm interested in what you're suggesting, but I need a little time to think about it."
2. *Speak from the heart* so it comes across as sincere and is less likely to sound like personal rejection.
3. *Ask about your partner's feelings and express your own* to open the door for an empowering conversation about the topic. Both of you will feel heard.

Care, Give, and Ask

At this point, any sex you're having with your partner has become more associative, connected, and embodied versus dissociated, disconnected, and mechanical. You are friendly lovers who care about and take care of each other. You give generously and receive well. You remember that you are responsible for your own sexual experiences, including your orgasms. You don't expect your partner to be a mind reader who's responsible for figuring out what you want and need. You don't take your partner's sexual preferences as a personal affront.

Instead, you talk about what *you* like and need. For example, if you're female and not lubricated enough, tell your partner so you don't have sex in silent discomfort. Such a scenario only leads to resentment. Make sure you have the lubrication you like at your bedside and use it freely, without shame. This is what real-time adult sexuality requires, unlike the sexuality promoted in movies and romance novels where no one bothers with such communication.

Don't forget to ask for oral sex. Oral sex can be a wonderful alternative to intercourse because there's no pressure involved to perform—just the receiving of pleasure. The act of oral sex allows you the experience of being in both the giving and receiving positions. If you don't like oral sex or being either the giver or receiver, I recommend that you ask yourself why. If your partner had oral sex with prostitutes and oral sex has become aversive to you as a result, talk about it. Express your feelings and consider how and if you can heal your aversion. If you can't come to a resolution with your partner, you may need more in-depth conversations with a therapist.

Often people don't like oral sex because they are uncomfortable with their own taste or the taste of their partner. Take time to talk about this with each other. Experiment with tasting your own sexual fluids and your partner's. Don't force oral sex on your partner. Instead, explore with each other doing things like bathing together and playing with flavored lubricants. This is another one of those times that may seem awkward or odd because it's so deliberate or conscious. In order for sex to take off in erotic and spontaneous ways, you have to be deliberate and explicit first. Power and control play out in all aspects of sexuality; giving is often the controlling position while receiving is the vulnerable position. Which position do you avoid and what do you know about your avoidance?

If you're male and your erection fails you, don't blame your partner or collapse into shame. Instead, enlist your partner's participation to get aroused. If your partner's erection fails, don't invent any stories about you doing something wrong or not being attractive or sexy enough.

At this stage of honesty and connection, hold on tight and stay true to yourself. Affirm that you are perfect, whole, and complete—for both you and your partner.

Find Happiness Through Connection

What part does happiness play in your ability to experience intimate, erotic sex with your partner? Your level of happiness gauges how well you're communicating and interacting with each other. When you've been through the painful, fearful times that make you question your abilities and emerge victorious, a remarkable growth takes place. Your inner resilience—the fire within you—becomes your strength and makes you far happier than having a high IQ, loads of money, or years of education. Happiness comes from your best, most challenging moments.

People who demonstrate happiness have strong ties to family and friends. Your commitment to each other adds to your happiness and can be further enhanced by your activities together. Having sex, relaxing, or engaging in spiritual practices together empowers couples to feel supported and safe, which equates to happiness. In the end, happiness is about your ability to connect with yourself and your partner, and to give and receive with a pure heart and clear intention. Your interpersonal engagement, whether in pillow talk, hot sex, or conversation over a cup of hot chocolate, is your key to success, as you've known throughout your recovery stages. Keep up the kindness and gratitude!

Move into Erotic Sex

As you move from intimate sex into erotic sex, remember that you include each facet of learning from previous chapters and then add to that experience. The new stage includes and transcends the previous one, creating richness, texture, and depth to your life story. Engaging in intimate sex, you're no longer hiding out and fantasizing about others. You have become fully present with yourself and your partner, preparing for your journey into the erotic.

Trust and commitment are essential for intimate sex, and orgasm is not a measure of your self-worth. From this vantage point, you learn that surrender and unleashing passion make for erotic sex.

What Is Erotic?

The term "erotic" conjures up different images in different people's minds, and those images change by gender, age, and personal experiences. "Erotic" refers to the intention to arouse sexual desire in oneself and the other. "Arouse" is active; therefore, erotic translates into actions and insinuations that can be subtle and either solitary or shared. Sex becomes erotic when one loses oneself in a loving connection with another person. It's this loving connection that transforms a common sex act into an erotic experience. As a result, the people involved are changed and affirmed.

Being erotic involves:

• Allowing passion
• Imagining
• Conversing
• Flirting
• Touching
• Planning and engaging in ritual
• Gazing into each other's eyes

The actions that you consider erotic are unique to you and your partner's experiences. I think of "eroticism" as a vital, pulsing energy in the body that longs to create and connect, like a live electrical wire flopping around loose after a disconnection. The live wire moves frenetically because the pulse dances in it. When it's reconnected to the correct charge, it finds a home. The no-longer-frenetic flow smooths out and feeds the connection.

So from my perspective, eroticism is:

• Connecting
• Dancing
• Pulsing
• Flowing
• Reconnecting
• Harmonizing

When Is the Right Time?

Erotic sex happens when both people become self-differentiated, meaning you've taken a stand for who you are sexually, are clear about it, and have revealed it to your partner. You and your partner have had conscious conversations and have been honest with each other about your feelings and your preferred sexual acts.

Chapter 1 defined "differentiation" as the balance between individuality and togetherness. As you move toward erotic sex, you make the commitment to comfort your anxieties. You're relaxed and not driven by fear of abandonment or, conversely, fear of being smothered and dependent.

It's important to embody the following states of being before you proceed:

• You can genuinely connect with each other.
• You no longer lose yourself to the relationship or act out your sexual desires with others.
• You own your sexuality and make yourself vulnerable by sharing it with your partner.
• You remain separate individuals in your personal truths while merging your energies through the most intimate act in which two people can engage.

Erotic sex allows a freedom to unleash the ravenous self while staying relational. That means when you're lost in the details of your experience, you're in the jet stream of eroticism, whether you're examining your partner's eyes or genitalia, or experimenting with the pace and rhythm of licking, sucking, or thrusting.

What Being Erotic Means
in a Relationship

What is being erotic like in a relationship? Here's what other couples have shared in answer to this question:

- "I watch my partner watch me during the sexual act, and it arouses me. We experience carnal pleasure and stay connected through eye contact."
- "In the beginning it was difficult for me to verbally express my feelings of love for my wife during sex. I had to tell myself it would be okay, then I took a leap of faith. At first I blurted the words out. My wife responded in a gentle and appreciative way. It's gotten easier over time, and now I love telling her I love her while I'm making love to her."
- "After we worked through being self-conscious, we let our animal passions come out. We accept the animal in totality and trust that a spiritual connection will grow out of that expression."

Eroticism Flows with Sexual Honesty

Eroticism happens more easily when you honor what is sexually true for you. That contrasts with being dishonorable when in sexual addiction. Now is the time to redeem your dignity. That means don't have sex if you don't want to; indeed, doing so could trigger going into fantasy, dissociating, or acting out sexually with your partner.

However, while moving into eroticism with your partner, it's crucial to ask yourself when you say no if you're saying no because you're hiding out. Maybe you don't want to deal with the discomfort of changing. In that case, the appropriate mind-set is to take responsibility by challenging yourself with rigorous honesty. Also talk with your partner about your discomfort so that both of you can better understand each other. Taking this approach develops a connection and allows for empathy.

When you take a good, deep look at yourself, you know that you will have to come to terms with how you create separation by judging your partner. You will also have to accept that the "frog" you married *is* your prince or princess. Any fantasies you've held on to about the "ideal one" must die and, as an adult, you must grieve that loss. The fact that your partner has "warts" doesn't make him or her any less perfect—only real. So believe that you are married to the perfect person, warts and all.

When you move into acceptance, you admit that your partner is separate from you, with different likes and dislikes. Can you see him or her as a separate sexual being, yet the two of you as a family? In this scenario, your disappointments and losses will surface. Let yourself grieve the loss of your fantasies, then move into gratitude for what you do have. The closer you get to your partner and the more deeply you connect during sex, the more deeply you will come to love.

Here's when a paradox arises. You have to hold on to the self you've worked so hard to develop in recovery and through the work in this book *while* merging with your partner during sex. This simple but not easy act creates a space for highly erotic sex to happen. When you reveal your most vulnerable self while staying emotionally connected, you can unleash your animalistic, carnal desires. The result is an experience of deep love, a different way of knowing yourself, and hot sex all at once!

Charlene and George's Story

In therapy, Charlene talked about her sexual discomfort with her husband, George, as their lovemaking moved from intimate to erotic. During the intimate stage, she and George shared how much they loved each other and were present for each other. But when sex moved beyond the comfortable, intimate stage into the erotic, Charlene had flashes of the pornographic images George used to watch online. These images seemed emblazoned in her mind; she simply couldn't shake them.

I explained to her that the images had burned themselves into her memory because they were novel and powerful. The brain loves novelty, and her reward-seeking neural networks grabbed on to those images so well, she couldn't shake them.

Why did these images pop up for Charlene during intercourse? When we examined this issue closely, she admitted that she would mentally leave during erotic sex with George because she felt uncomfortable. On the one hand, she was extremely turned on and wanted to express her full-on sexuality with him. On the other, her discomfort hung on the edge of increasing her love for George, yet she was too afraid to go there completely. Loving and trusting George brought up the fear that she could experience the pain of betrayal all over again. What if George acted out sexually in the future? What would happen if she released those feelings with George during sex instead of switching to the pornographic images?

Charlene's next step was to risk shedding her tears—all mixed with love, anger, and fear—with George. By talking it out, both of them realized that everything she felt was normal, especially in clearing the way for erotic sex.

George's role during sex was to have empathy for his wife, hold her tightly, keep his penis inside her, and not get defensive and abandon her due to his shame. He was instructed not to take her feelings personally. To honor her and himself in this way would be tender and could lead to a more profound sexual experience between them.

As a couple, George and Charlene learned to tolerate their discomfort in order to experience the depth of connection created by truly looking into each other. When they looked, they were willing to feel their own pain and also the power of their love. In that moment, their sex became a prayer for healing.

Couples like them will connect in a new way when they can answer these crucial questions in the affirmative:

- Can Charlene handle her animal nature without naming it "pornographic"?
- Can she remind herself of who she is, not the damaged, sleazy woman imagined in the porn but a vital, alive, desirous woman?
- Does she believe that her husband can see her for who she is and not mistake her for something dirty?
- Can she allow her heart to open, knowing the perils that lie ahead?
- Can he stay in his integrity and not mislead or lie to his wife again?
- Can they each accept the other's vulnerabilities?
- Can they both face the discomfort that comes with the call to love each other more deeply?

What If the Flow Ebbs?

When you're connected to your partner, eroticism ebbs and flows. You *invite* eroticism because you can't corral or own it. Eroticism arrives as a result of the intentions you have set, your willingness to be open, and your desire to know yourself and your partner more deeply. Eroticism has its own rhythms and seasons. Given that, you'll have times when you feel wildly in love with your partner and grateful you sustained your partnership. You'll also have times when you hardly give him or her a second thought. When the flow ebbs, remember that the intimate sex we talked about in Chapter 7 can be different but just as satisfying as the erotic sex discussed here. So be mindful and know that if you stay aware in the ways we've been working toward, the erotic feelings will return and visit you again and again.

Accept Reality; Show Trust

Love is immensely fulfilling, yet it also inherently involves losses. We have to accept that. Marriage is *not* a bliss trip. Rather, it's the constant pursuit of change, growth, and the ability to deeply love— and it requires admitting that you *can't* have it all.

Grief and love become inextricably bound together as you admit to yourself who you are and who your partner is, and that your body is changing, your looks are fading, your children are aging, and your parents are dying. Moving into your eroticism as an adult requires a reality check, because you have to let the fantasy of storybook love and movielike sex die. On the other hand, adult eroticism allows for ongoing exploration of what love means to you and who you are sexually.

When you have trust as a couple, anything goes. Conversely, if any feelings of betrayal still linger in your partnership, you don't have a green light to move forward. What happens when fear, pain, or anger arise from your partner about your sex with others, or when past sexual abuse memories come up during sex? Talking with your partner about these can be a powerful healing force, allowing you to work through your issues as part of your erotic exploration. If such conversations are difficult, you can always seek assistance from a qualified therapist.

Grow Spiritually Through Sex

Erotic sex emerges when you engage *totally* with your partner—and the deeper your connection, the more profound your spiritual feelings will be.

To move toward spiritual sex, any role of victimhood must fade away so you can admit to yourself that you're in your relationship voluntarily. You take full responsibility for being in your relationship, ready to hold your center while surrendering to the unknown, where you continue to discover your sexuality, your partner, and your relationship with the divine (you'll find out more about the spiritual aspect of sex in Chapter 11).

✓ Erotic Intelligence Checklist for Chapter 8

❏ Three aspects vital to maintaining a positive connection with yourself and your partner are: (1) being able to say no, meaning it, and having your boundaries respected; (2) saying yes, being heard, and following through; and (3) offering an alternate plan if the one that's being presented to you is not right in the moment.

❏ Three keys to honest pillow talk that will leave both of you feeling heard and loved, rather than ignored and blamed are: (1) using the language of "I" statements; (2) speaking from the heart; and (3) asking about your partner's feelings and expressing your own.

❏ Moving into your eroticism as an adult requires a reality check because you have to let the fantasy of storybook love and movielike sex die. On the other hand, adult eroticism allows for ongoing exploration of what love means to you and who you are sexually.

9

The Essence of Eroticism

---

*No matter how familiar we are with
each other, with our surroundings, we cannot
get bored if we truly pay attention.*

—Philip T. Sudo (1959–)

Undifferentiated people express boredom with each other in a relationship due to the rigidity of their ways and lack of willingness to deal with conflict in order to grow and change. In contrast, *differentiated* people are willing to live in the world of the unknown because they challenge themselves to tell the truth about who they really are. To do this, they need to pay attention.

As emphasized earlier, truth telling facilitates your growth and change on an ongoing basis, both personally and sexually. Defining eroticism becomes part of your ever-changing process. So set your intention to be erotic and trust that every sexual encounter you have will clarify and expand your definition.

Dance a New Dance

Chapter 1 described the metaphor of the dance of intimacy and sexuality. By now, you're "dancing" together, taking turns leading and following. But what are some fine points when choreographing this new dance? Here are a few suggestions.

Accept your differences and relax. That's when the mysteries of sex will be revealed to you. You're in this relationship to love, support, give, receive, challenge and evoke new and exciting dimensions for each other. At this juncture in your journey, sex is no longer energy draining and depressing, as it was in your sexually addictive past. Instead, it's become life affirming.

Let patience be your guide and follow your heart. The erotic energy you're patiently creating is composed of your bodies merging, touching, caressing, kissing, and reaching toward each other as you fall together and apart, merging and diverging.

Begin your foreplay before you get to the bedroom. Foreplay can start several days before you have sex. You can call your partner and leave provocative messages or write e-mails with sexual innuendos that evoke a sense of play (if privacy can be assured).

Take time to connect personally. Talk to each other about how you're feeling and what you need. Look deeply into each other's eyes, hold hands, stroke his face, touch her hair, and take time for subtle kisses. Share your favorite foods and make each other laugh. Bring all of who you are to the fore to seduce and arouse your partner.

Delight your partner with small surprises. Bring home bright flowers, spicy take-out food, or a sweet square of dark Belgian chocolate.

Plan your sexual trysts. Don't resist the idea of planning sex. Doing so allows you to set an intention and begin the titillation of anticipation.

Be deliberate and thoughtful in your seduction. Eroticism begins with the intention behind how you interact with your partner.

Allow Nervous Excitement to Show

Whether you're scared or excited, talk about what you're feeling every step of the way. Listen to what your partner reports and don't judge it; just listen. It's okay to be scared and go forward anyway; it's the process of learning to trust. You made a decision to stay in the relationship, so remind yourself to be responsible for your choices.

Adults manage their discomfort and tension about sex because they understand that's where arousal comes from. Sometimes anxiety and excitement can feel the same. Don't try to get rid of your feelings; instead, *lean into them* so you can have the experience of settling yourself down. By calming your nervous excitement, you will have a new sexual experience and "cut new grooves."

During your addiction, sex had become a numbers game, a function of chasing novelty to stimulate the brain and rid yourself of anxiety. But sex is now about inviting a kind of nervous excitement, not rushing to cover it up or push it away. Accept that part of your adult sexuality and recognize it as the engine that arouses you and your partner. Revel in the arousal. Pay attention. Keep your eyes open, noticing what you see and how you feel. If shame arises, work with it by calming yourself down with positive self-talk. If the shame becomes too overwhelming, stop what you're doing.

Know that you can accept your feelings without judgment. It's okay to show your discomfort, awkwardness, and vulnerability with your partner. You won't always look cool or smooth, but you'll be authentic and real. Take responsibility for the feelings by allowing them and talking to your partner as they come up. This openness is what it means to really get naked while this kind of honesty will deepen the connection between the two of you, bringing you closer so you can love more deeply.

Above all, have compassion for yourself and empathy for your partner. You might be surprised to find that once the pain subsides, your sexual desire for your partner increases. Why? Because being seen and heard is a powerful aphrodisiac. It's time to proceed confidently from this place of increased vulnerability, realizing that you've just struck gold!

Create Special Symbols and Spaces

What symbols have meaning to you as a couple? What items make your sexual intention tangible? Many couples have chosen a stone, a cross, a candle, a small Buddha statue, a poem, a Star of David, or a nature scene. Think of the erotic as a creative force. Design an inspiring space for creativity and honesty to flow. Think about what you would add to your space that demonstrates empathy for your partner. Determine what would have your partner feeling more trusting and comfortable as you move toward eroticism together.

Stimulate Your Senses

Evoking the five senses helps stimulate the entire body and bring your lovemaking to a more pleasurable level. Let's look at how each sense can play a part.

Lauren and Joan's Story

Six months into their recovery, Lauren and Joan created an altar in their bedroom as a place where they could remember and relish their journey together. They used the altar as a symbol of their fifteen years together and to commemorate Lauren's sobriety. They chose photos of happy times and of their parents and children. Lauren placed small symbols of her recovery on the altar. Joan added her airline stub from her visit to Lauren during the treatment program's family week. On days when they planned to have sex, they added a simple flower to represent a new beginning. They also placed water for purity of heart and a small bowl of rice symbolizing the proliferation of life.

Sight

The eyes have been called the windows to the soul, which can also explain why gazing into each other's eyes deepens and enhances your sexual experience.

In addition, eyes serve to connect the brain and body with the outer world. Humans are visual creatures who look at anything that moves or catches the eye. Because our brains are stimulated by what we see, the more novel something appears, the more interesting and arousing it is to both the brain and body. This explains, in part, why we're curious about anything new.

The nerves in the eye connect to both the central nervous system and the autonomic nervous system, acting as "periscopes" for the brain and body. This contributes to stimulating sexual arousal.

To make your erotic sex more appealing visually, have a conversation with your partner about what stimulates you both visually and why. My suggestions include making eye contact during sex, watching each other undress or slowly undressing each other, softening the lighting, or even using candles.

You can determine which colors appeal to each of you and use color in your sex play. Years of research by Dr. Max Lüscher inform us that color affects behavior. His studies show that the characteristics of certain colors "can be used to measure your erotic/love experience and to discover your romantic self." For example, purple relates to devotion and bonding, magenta creates a feeling of resonance to yourself and the other, orange is equated with sexual arousal, and cinnamon pink the desire for fantasies and expectations.[1] What's your favorite color? What's your lover's favorite color? Get creative about how you use that information.

In addition, the clothing you wear can be sexually stimulating, which is obvious from the fashion ads that surround us. If you know your partner finds you attractive in a certain color or article of clothing, why not dress to make yourself *feel* more attractive so your partner will see you as attractive?

Sound

After visual cues, sound is the second most arousing sexual experience for men. Most men consider the satisfied sounds their partners make during sex to be a fantastic aphrodisiac. Pleasurable sounds during sex heighten the experience, especially if paired with imagery that also pleasures you. In his book *Great Sex*, Michael Castleman suggests that deep sighs and low moans—resonances of sexual pleasures—are contagious because sounds coming from the emotional, primitive part of the brain send arousal signals to your partner.[2]

Too often, people keep the sounds of their own pleasure silent or censor the sounds, bottling up their sexual energy. This is a time to allow *you* to come forward. When exhaling, let yourself sigh deeply, and allow yourself to speak sexually charged words. Doing this moves energy at a high velocity, which is what our bodies are designed to do. If you bottle up the energy, you may be left feeling unsatisfied.

Studies show that the use of strong sexual language during sex can further amplify the intensity of sexual pleasure. Sexual sounds are a language used to transmit information to each other without using speech. However, both males and females experienced sounds as positive, wanted their partners to make them, and believed them to be signals of sexual satisfaction. When females direct males with verbal instructions like "deeper, harder, faster," males find this highly arousing. Likewise, female vocalizations during sex intensify more than those of males do as the male moves toward orgasm. Females are more aroused by touch and music than males.[3]

Consider these options for enhancing your sexual pleasure through sounds:

• Make your own natural sounds of pleasure: groaning, grunting, humming, or sighing.
• Listen to each other's breathing.
• Whisper to each other words that arouse you: "I cherish you"; "You are sexy and beautiful"; "You feel so good inside me."
• Choose music you both enjoy or select natural sounds like a waterfall, the wind, or the ocean to relax you.

Taste and Smell

Taste and smell are intertwined sensory modalities for stimulating pleasures and creating fragrant memories. For example, dark chocolate balances serotonin and dopamine levels and provides sweet tastiness. Fruits can be juicy snacks that you put at your bedside to share before, during, and after sex.

Smell can be an aphrodisiac for many people. Go shopping together for aromatic body oils that you love smelling on your partner's skin, and use them on your bodies prior to or during sex. Whether you use oils or prefer the natural scents of your bodies, remember to attend to your personal hygiene. Showering, shaving, and brushing your teeth make you a more appealing lover. Of course, showering or bathing *together* with soothing, warm water heightens your sensuality.

Personal hygiene is especially important to women. Women's genitals produce a number of different secretions and odors, from pheromones to sexual lubrication, to blood. Though some women are shamed about it, comedians joke about it, and commercial products abound to sanitize female odor away, many men and women are sexually stimulated by the smell of natural secretions.

Scented candles, flowers, and clean linens all add to the sensual orgy of arousal. However, it's best to discuss personal preferences in perfumes and colognes before putting them on. Share what you like and don't like, how much is enough, and how much is too much.

Pheromones are chemical substances produced by an animal or an insect. The most important source of pheromones in humans is the skin. Our capacity to sniff out a mate is uncanny, and a person's scent can make a difference in whether or not we find someone attractive. Animals secrete pheromones into the environment to cause a behavioral change in other animals. According to a study at San Francisco State University, pheromones on humans evoke kissing or petting.[4] How? In this study, researchers tested a perfume laced with synthetic pheromones, which increased the women's sexual attractiveness to men. (Men, in pheromone

studies, your cologne didn't do much to arouse women's interests!)
The study also found these results:

• Men prefer pumpkin and lavender odors.
• Women prefer the scent of almond.
• The scent of cherry increases blood flow by 13 percent in
  women.

So find out if he enjoys a foot massage, then provide one using
light massage oil with a pumpkin scent. Perhaps she likes a bubble
bath. If so, run the hot water and pour in almond bath crystals. But
don't stop there. Use your imaginations. Experiment with different
scents you find and give them to each other as gifts. Combine scents
that appeal to you or try adding aphrodisiac foods, such as bananas,
nuts, cucumbers, cherries, pumpkin pie, and so on into your foreplay.[5]

Touch

Touching each other is a major element of erotica. Why? Touch
pleasures us by releasing the chemical oxytocin, causing us to desire
more. Oxytocin sets up a feedback loop of touching, pleasure, and
further desire to be touched and pleasured.

When women are touched, the chemical combination of oxytocin
and estrogen enhances enjoyable responses, such as the sensitivity
of nipples and genitalia to stimulation. Reaching orgasm invigorates
her desires even more. These pleasurable hormonal reactions help
couples forget that they argued, felt pain, or had conflict. Touching
and hugging promote erotic feelings, and on a basic biochemical
level, human beings need touch in order to thrive.

Often in relationships where the man is recovering from sex addiction, the woman feels deprived of touch by her partner. The sex
addict, because of his shame or difficulties with intimacy, does not

experience touching his partner as second nature. If you feel uncomfortable cuddling, touching, or showing physical affection with the woman in your life, now is the time to stretch yourself and begin the exploration. Notice where you feel discomfort in your body. Breathe and stay with your feelings as you focus on your partner. What does touch evoke in you? Why are you so uncomfortable? Remember, females find touch both sexually arousing and pleasing; touch gives them the feeling they are loved and cared for.

Simple Methods of Touch

If you and your partner need to train yourselves to consciously touch each other, consider these simple methods that promote biochemical and psychological connection:

- Hold hands during a movie.
- Enjoy full-body hugs, engaging heart to heart and pelvis to pelvis.
- Walk arm in arm.
- Sit close together, touching.
- Snuggle in bed.
- Give each other neck and shoulder massages.

Kissing

Kissing is an erotic act. Many people tell me they don't like kissing but haven't examined why. Some say they wish their partners would forget about it. *But if you aspire to erotic sex, give up the idea that you don't have to address your inadequacies or that your partner should let you off the hook.* If the problem is something simple to rectify, like your partner's breath, then you both need to talk and find out what to change. Don't take a complaint like bad breath lightly. If you aren't willing to address your bad breath, then you're probably not talking about what's really going on with you. Ask yourself, "Why am I throwing up a roadblock to being sexual?"

Did you know that rejecting kissing is a way of rejecting yourself? Many people don't like kissing because it's too much closeness. Sex addicts can have sex with strangers, but connecting closely with their loved one becomes uncomfortable, and kissing brings you close. It's about feeling and being felt. Kissing arouses your body, if you allow it, signaling that you're aroused by the other person. Tasting your partner, exchanging saliva, and feeling the scent and heat of your partner's breath can be arousing if shame is not in the way. When you give yourself over to the sensations that arise from kissing your lover, you'll find your thoughts cease.

Kissing is another kind of dance in which moving slowly is erotic and licking quickly can cause orgasm. Try nibbling, flicking your tongue, licking slowly, biting gently, and giving soft kisses and deeper, longer ones. Let your partner know what you like best while exploring the deep arousal that kissing can bring.

Remember, you can't *get* or *give* too much touch, which is essential in eroticism. Touch enhances the act of kissing and creates further arousal. Once you get into bed, take your time to stimulate your partner's body erotically. Touch his or her hands, arms, neck, fingers, toes, calves, and thighs. Let your partner know where you most like to be touched. Some people like to be softly tickled, while others love to have their back scratched or massaged, for example. Take a trip to the exotic landscape of your lover's body and learn about your erogenous zones together. Your intent is to give up control *and* be in service of the other.

Masturbation

Direct your partner in exactly how you'd like to be touched so you can reach your optimal level of arousal. Teach your partner how you'd like to be masturbated. Show what points on your penis or clitoris are most sensitive.

For most women, clitoral orgasms are easier to have than vaginal ones. However, be mindful that the clitoris is more sensitive than the head of the penis. So if you want to have more vaginal orgasms, take time to learn about your G-spot and educate your partner about where to find it. Typically, it's a few inches inside on the upper wall of the vagina. But if you need more information, instructional media on the topic are available.

Let your partner watch you masturbate and notice how you feel being watched as you make eye contact. Experience what it's like to be seen and loved as you express your sexuality. How does it feel to arouse your partner? Heighten your awareness. Next time you masturbate in front of your partner, let him or her take over. Use your hands on top of your partner's as you guide him or her toward the kind of pressure and rhythm you like best. Feel free to use lubrication and give instructions about the pace and rhythm that pleasures you. Be on the lookout for shame, which might arrive uninvited. Remember who's in control; just gently ask the shame to leave.

Pace Yourself

In erotic sex, slowing down is critical to allow time for reveling in all the senses and connecting emotionally on a deep level. In addition, a slow pace during sex keeps the entire body stimulated rather than going for brain stimulation, the dopamine surge, and getting off. A slowed-down pace calms anxiety and can help prevent erectile dysfunction and rapid ejaculation. In addition, it's crucial for a man to understand he must slow to a women's pace. Women love the feeling of sexual anticipation, so slow down. Your instinct may be to carry her off to the bedroom, but try a long make-out session on the sofa instead. As you slow down, the female sexual excitation system will interpret colors, sights, sounds, and scents as hotly erotic. At this point, take time to touch her with a light touch. (Guys, your touch is 20 percent more forceful than hers, so be sensitive to that.) Try areas that don't get touched often, such as the underside of her arms, her collarbone, and areas around her breasts. As you slow your pace, her arousal will increase, and she will respond by moving toward you, signaling you for more.

Bust the Myths

Most myths that fill our culture need to be actively combated. Pornography, for one, ignores the truth about real women and men. Women's needs are mythologized, turning women into objects that are all the same. How far that is from the truth! Women are not interchangeable sex objects without their own, unique needs. Most require a period of foreplay to warm up before having sex, so they're not "at the ready" the minute a man shows up with an erection.

Let's recognize that men are also treated as objects in the world of pornography. Many men report the desire to connect first before being sexual; they enjoy being seen, valued, and touched. Contrary to popular myths, they don't all have unnaturally large penises that are always erect.

Remember, erotic anticipation has to build. Partners of sex addicts often feel inadequate, stating that they "can't compete with outside images of sex," or don't think they'll "ever measure up." No one looks like the people they see in porn scenes because those bodies are either really young, have been reconstructed through plastic surgery, or are airbrushed after filming. So stop comparing yourself and your partner to those images. Be respectful of your partner's needs and factor that into the equation of how to set the sexual stage.

Talk Sexually

Sex addicts worry about talking sexually, fearing that their partners will think they want them to re-create their acting-out trysts. Their partners worry that sexual talk will trigger the addicts into their old behaviors. As a result, both parties keep silent, which limits their eroticism.

Yet due to the recovery work you've done, you *can be relational* with your partner. You are making the choice to *connect* in profound ways, not to simply arouse your body without context. All the work you've done thus far to reveal yourselves to each other should have you feeling more confident and clear about who you are and what you want. You're involved in an ongoing growth process that requires conscious, deliberate, and lively communication—so speak up about your sexual desires. Erotic talk whispered into your lover's ear can set more than the soul on fire.

Express your carnal desire, what you're seeing, and what you'd like to see or do with your partner, whether it is lovely, lustful, or lascivious. This kind of connection ignites your partner's physical arousal as well as your own.

However, if sex talk has been part of your acting out with your partner, then refrain from it until you have examined it fully. Remember, you can act out sexually in a relationship as much as you can with a stranger if you're not mindful.

Shawn and Jennifer's Story

Shawn and Jennifer had been married for twelve years. While Shawn was in his addiction, they both relied on sex talk and fantasy as a matter of course during sex together. Both agreed that they *needed* the sex talk and fantasy in order to get aroused. That's because they were both in their own separate worlds, arousing their brains, not their hearts.

Jennifer didn't know Shawn was having affairs, but she did know about his fantasy of imagining her having sex with another man while he watched. This fantasy, although arousing to both of them, took them *out* of connection with each another. Jennifer kept her eyes closed and focused on the fantasy and sensations in her body while shutting Shawn out. Shawn would objectify Jennifer's body parts without making any kind of heart connection with her. In fact, he was solely interested in "getting off."

This style of sex might be okay on occasion, but with Shawn and Jennifer, it was the only way they could get to arousal with each other. Therefore, they needed to back up and start over again with healthy sex. Sex talk and fantasy of this nature became off-limits for them for some time.

Once Jennifer admitted her discomfort in getting too close to Shawn, it seemed fine to have sex with her eyes closed in fantasy. Having grown up with a domineering stepfather, complying with

Shawn's needs was what she thought she was supposed to do to keep him sexually happy. In all these years, she had never thought about her own sexuality or what truly aroused her or had meaning for her.

Shawn's history of engaging in power struggles preceded his marriage to Jennifer. In recovery, he came to understand that his habitual patterns with women stemmed from his mother's sadistic, emotional abuse of him as a child. He could never get anything right for her, and he eventually took his anger out on women in sexual escapades.

Shawn was most aroused when he became sadistic, ordering women around and engaging them sexually in anything that was humiliating or denigrating. That way, he could feel as if he was in control and had power in his life. Eventually, though, whoever he was involved with would catch him, and Shawn would revert to the child who was in trouble. He paid heavy consequences, usually losing his relationship. Yet playing the masochist was also arousing for him. Based on his history, Shawn believed he deserved to be punished. The cycle repeated itself until his last exploit nearly destroyed his marriage to Jennifer. That's when he decided it was time to change.

Sexual recovery demanded that Shawn be vulnerable and reveal these patterns to himself and to Jennifer. Eliminating degrading fantasy from his sex life with Jennifer meant he had to connect, which made him uncomfortable. Not surprisingly, he felt vulnerable having to trust a woman, give up control, and tolerate receiving pleasure and being watched.

At the same time, Jennifer had to stop hiding behind her little girl patterns and come forward with her sexuality as a grown woman.

She also had to stop worrying about what she *should* do to ensure arousing Shawn. Rather, her focus as an adult was on what aroused her, trusting that if she became honest about her own desires, she would arouse Shawn.

Feelings After Sex

People in recovery experience a wide variety of feelings during and after having sex. These feelings may vary from satisfaction and fulfillment to sadness or loneliness. No one feeling is better than or more appropriate than the other. They are what they are.

I suggest you check in with yourself after having sex and ask these questions:

- What do you need?
- Do you want to cuddle closer and feel your partner's heartbeat?
- Do you need to face each other and breathe together?
- Do you need to cry and talk about what came up for you as your partner patiently listens without judgment?
- Are you feeling chatty and elated?
- Do you feel like talking or making a yummy snack afterward?

Because each sexual encounter is different, resist expectations and doing things in a predictable, rote way. Remember, sex is never a *thing* you just had. Sex is the intercourse, the merging or convergence, of who the two of you are—your spirits merging.

People ask, "How was *it* for you?" The reply is often, "*It* was great." But is this really the right question and answer? Instead, personalize your question and ask, "How are you?" Respond with depth. Gaze into each other's eyes and speak your truth: "I'm over the moon," or "I love you," or "I melted and I'm just coming back into myself." *There are no wrong answers!*

Allow Connection and Healing

The Four Cornerstones of Intimacy repeatedly appear as part of the process of coming together through opening up, loving, and remaining willing to bare your feelings and truths. Because of your willingness to *reveal* yourself and *accept* your partner with no judgments or opinions, your connection opens the door to your heart's thoughtful simplicity. *Responsibility* says that you are an adult who can hold your center, remain present with your partner, and focus your intentions together to create your lifestyle and love style. *Empathy* allows the hurt, lost, or confused parts of you to merge into a person who can engage in healthy, erotic sex as an adult.

Turn to the Four Cornerstones again—self-knowledge, comfort and connection, responsibility with discernment, empathy with emotion—to reestablish the healing and connection you seek.

Create Your Own Story for Erotic Sex

At this point in your sexual journey, your purpose in creating desire in yourself and in each other is to ignite arousal and initiate sex. So if you were orchestrating a seductive, romantic evening with your partner for hot sex, how would you write this part of your story?

I suggest you start by asking yourself these questions:

• What romantic ploys does your partner enjoy?
• How does he or she like to be seduced?

- How do you like to flirt?
- What makes you feel desirable?
- What touch, smile, or other innuendos do you use?

Sex addicts use a lot of this behavior with others to get to orgasm (and dopamine) or to control others, but shame keeps them from doing it in a present, vulnerable, deliberate, conscious way with their partners. When you're writing your story to please your partner, feel free to be wildly creative!

✓ Erotic Intelligence Checklist for Chapter 9

❑ Set the erotic stage by stimulating all five senses.

❑ Invite a kind of nervous excitement into your sex life, recognizing it as the engine that arouses you and your partner.

❑ Express your carnal desire, which includes what you're smelling, tasting, touching, hearing, and especially what you'd like to do with your partner.

Role-Playing and Sexual Fantasy

---

*Sexual fantasies may call forth new life
in the guise of new sexual experiences, and
so the motive for repressing these fantasies may
not be as much moral sensitivity as fear
of life's irrepressible abundance.*

—Thomas Moore (1940–)

Erotica happens when you've self-differentiated, you're allowing your heart and soul to be your guides, and you and your partner resonate as one. At this stage, role-playing can be delightful when the use of fantasy includes each other. Fantasy is healthy, especially now that you and your partner have learned to trust yourselves and each other. Remember, healthy sex means fantasy does *not* involve shame, abuse to yourself or your partner, avoidance of feelings, or emotional disconnection from your partner. While fantasy in sex addiction is often used to deny and avoid past trauma, *healthy* fantasy can serve to more deeply connect you and your partner.

Because sexuality is so complex, this is not a one-size-fits-all proposition and may not work for all recovering couples. If your forays into healthy fantasy with your partner has you dissociating or drifting into the euphoric recall of past sexual experiences, consider that this activity may not right for you. Stop. Return to Chapter 9 and stay with a more directly connected, sensual approach to your sexuality. Take your concerns into your therapy sessions.

Try on New Sexual Roles

Trying new sexual roles in relational sexual activities is not for everyone. If you try it and discover it has value for you and your partner, then get clear about what makes you feel sexy and desirable and let your partner know. This goes well beyond pillow talk!

If dressing up sexually is fun for you, do it! Some people like to be looked at in sexual ways taking on various roles, finding this form of sex play highly erotic. Have a conversation with your partner about what makes each of you nervous or excited in this arena.

For example, some addicts who were once part of a "leather scene," and who wish to restore their sexuality after a compulsive lifestyle, may still find themselves turned on by leather. If that applies to you, how do you engage your fetish with leather without exploiting yourself or your partner? Can you do it in private with your partner and not in the exhibitionist way you may have done it in the past? As always, your goal is to hold on to the loving connection between you and your partner.

Some women like to wear lacy lingerie, jewelry, provocative clothing, and other baubles or use heavier makeup than they do during their workday. It's because dressing up makes them feel sexual and alive. It turns them on to enjoy hot sex, not solely to generate a sense of power and control over their partners.

Do you enjoy elaborate costumes or rituals that involve the enticing anticipation of undressing? Or do you tend to play dominant or submissive roles while having sex? If so, make sure you are far enough along in your recovery to do this with respect.

Shawn and Jennifer's Story

When Shawn and Jennifer (Chapter 9) first met, they had instant chemistry between them; he liked being sexually dominant and she liked being sexually submissive. In his addiction, Shawn would act out the role of the dominant male in a way that made him feel powerful both with other women and with Jennifer. He would also act out his unconscious rage at women, ordering Jennifer around during sex in denigrating ways. Although she found this kind of sex physically arousing, it also left her feeling lonely and bad about herself.

After Shawn admitted he had a problem with addiction, they both went into recovery. Their sexual healing included Jennifer becoming more her own person. Shawn dealt with his discomfort around giving up control, receiving pleasure, and being overtly loving. Once they put all the pieces together and became more integrated both individually and as a couple, they discovered they still liked their respective roles of domination and submission. What was the difference? Their sex was more relational—that is, Shawn and Jennifer were more present, honest, and alive with themselves and each other.

Sex can be dominant or submissive depending on what you are thinking during the sexual act itself. When giving oral sex, are you imagining yourself as being in control, "taking" your partner, or are you feeling submissive as if you are in "service" of your partner? These rhythms shift and change in sex, and when you are honest about them, you amplify your eroticism.

In Shawn and Jennifer's case, they began to allow for the organic shifts of domination and submission to happen but were able to stay connected with each other, making eye contact and saying "I love you" during the sexual act. Their "roles" were now more congruent with who they were individually and who they agreed they wanted to be as a couple. This subtle but important shift contrasted with their pre-recovery sex, which was more like two actors playing out their parts while disconnected and dissociated.

Jada and Rick's Story

Jada and Rick loved the heat of prolonging their sexual experiences whenever they could, but with three children and two busy careers, they barely had time for sex. On the occasions when Jada's sister took the kids for the evening, Rick and Jada turned their rare Saturday night dates into long lovemaking sessions. This luxury of time gave them the opportunity to slow down and luxuriate in each other.

Date nights sometimes started with dressing up, dining at a fine restaurant, lingering over dessert, and returning home for sumptuous sex. They set a mood of romantic mystique that began with a ritual of undressing each other, watching and slowly kissing and touching all the while. Rick, a music collector, compiled a CD of music with Brazilian rhythms that Jada danced to, while she tended to the details of fresh flowers, aromatherapy scents, and lighting. Then they brought out their sensual toys—feathers, silk scarves, and other objects they had previously agreed to use to be titillating.

Jada knew from their values list that a sense of adventure and novelty aroused Rick. She so delighted in her new sexuality, she felt restored after the destructive effects of Rick's sexual acting out had healed. Four years into recovery, she felt secure with herself and within their coupleship. Rick no longer needed contrived danger for intensity, such as seeking out dangerous sexual escapades via hookups on the Internet with strange women and sometimes men. He now found the qualities of adventure and novelty through his renewed relationship with Jada. Through his recovery and the work he and Jada have done together, he has healed a lot of his childhood trauma. More than that, he values himself and his sexuality and experiences Jada as new and exciting. Jada took risks to show and tell Rick who she was sexually. Together, they continue to be sexually adventurous and enjoy talking about what they discover.

Sensual toys, not necessarily sex toys, and sensual activities are fine if they're appropriate for you and your partner. Try using "toys" like feathers, silky fabrics, dusting powders, or washable body paints. Take hot baths together before or after you make love. Use your imagination to fantasize, but always clarify your boundaries. Pay attention to your partner's sexual and sensual cues. Be willing to say "yes" to invitations for intimacy or sex, but also don't be afraid to say or hear "no."

Play with Sexual Fantasy

Earlier, you reviewed the meaning of acting out your sexual fantasies in an attempt to examine what qualities or values you were seeking. In adult sexuality, you pay attention to your current fantasies, discuss them with your partner, and listen to his or hers without reaction or judgment. In a healthy relationship, your sexual fantasies keep desire alive as part of your endless search for understanding what sex means to you.

But be sure to monitor your fantasies. Everyone's mind wanders during sex. Accept this fact! The real question is *where* does your mind wander? Are you in euphoric recall of past sexual acting-out experiences? Do you harbor fantasies of a future experience with someone you wouldn't tell your partner about? If so, you're most likely in your addictive mind. Stop when those kinds of fantasies arise during sex with your partner. Collect yourself by breathing, looking deeply at your partner, and talking to him or her. Let your partner know you were drifting away, and then shift to staying connected. If this continues, creating fantasies may not be for you. Return to the erotic, sensual sex discussed in Chapter 9.

On the other hand, are you thinking about the kids or worried about work? Are you wondering when sex will be over? This kind of thinking also means you're not present with your partner. Both acting-out fantasies and mental wanderings are escapes from emotional connection with your partner.

Consider this alternative: Include your partner in your sexual fantasy. If you're fantasizing a scene that arouses you, share it with your partner. Telling your partner doesn't hurt him or her or exact revenge. The point is to have an honest conversation, without shame, about what's hot for you. People struggle with this difficult conversation because they're afraid their partner will become angry. And sometimes partners do get upset.

If you're on the receiving end in this situation, it may mean you're still relying on your partner to validate your worthiness and lovability, and you'll probably get angry. However, if you've done the work explained in this book, you've become more differentiated, so you won't collapse into shame or react to what your partner is saying. In fact, you won't be surprised to hear your partner say that images of other people are arousing because you'll probably admit the same is true for you. *The kind of risk taking that involves telling your truth directly will heat up your sex life.*

Remember that fantasy is just that. Not surprisingly, the most frequent erotic fantasy people report involves a different partner, and their fantasies are usually out of the realm of the reality of their sex lives.[1] Often people have sexual fantasies they would never act out. You'll tap into fantasies that include your partner and others you invent together to increase your erotic styles.

Jeanine and Art's Story

As a partner of a sex addict in recovery, Jeanine herself was in recovery and working on her own sexuality. As a young woman, she'd been repressed by a strict religious upbringing. Consequently, Jeanine never experienced varied sexual experimentation in her teens or twenties. She met Art when she was thirty, fell in love, and enjoyed the sex they had with each other without knowing why or what her sexual preferences were. Slowly her sexual desire dwindled without her understanding why. After they married, Art went back to his sex addiction. He was wounded by her disinterest and used it to justify having sex outside their marriage. But by going for sexual massages, he was living a double life. Between her low sexual desire and raising their two children, Jeanine still didn't pay much attention to her impoverished sex life with Art.

At forty-two, Jeanine and Art had been in recovery for three years when she realized—and admitted to herself—that the idea of Art watching her have sex with another woman turned her on. Jeanine didn't come to this realization overnight. She'd spent a lot of time in her personal therapy talking about her family issues and why she'd been so shut down sexually as a young woman. As she felt less shame about being a sexual being and got more in touch with her own sexual urges, Jeanine let herself fantasize about many sexual possibilities. Although she had never been with a woman and felt sure she never wanted to, the *idea* of it aroused her. She wanted to incorporate the fantasy into her sex life with Art, but first, she had to tell him without shame overtaking her.

Remembering that anxiety is a natural part of any new activity, she took a deep breath and told him directly. Art was uncomfortable hearing this from Jeanine, of all people, and he was confused about where it fit with his recovery. However, when he focused on Jeanine, this activity no longer triggered him. In fact, he felt delighted seeing her as a sexual being.

In bed one day, Jeanine took another risk and decided to tell Art she would like to create a fantasy with him, saying, "I was having lunch yesterday with a redheaded woman from my office. I saw you pass by on the other side of the street and noticed you looking at us."

Art picked up the story and said, "Yes, I saw you watching me notice the two of you."

Jeanine continued, "I pretended to drop my napkin on the ground, and when I reached down to pick it up, I brushed my hand along her calf as if it were an accident."

"I saw the woman blush and flinch as you touched her and wondered what you would do next. I was surprised!" Art added.

"She seemed flirtatious with me, so I kissed her cheek, all the while watching you, Art."

By then, their imaginations were off and running!

Jeanine and Art exemplify the point that it's important for you and your partner to build your sexual fantasies together, making them about and with each other. As a result, you'll have no secrets, shame, or abuse.

At the Threshold

When you're fully naked and vulnerable, sexual potential comes from surrendering—that is, from *not trying*. The moves and manipulations you turned to as a sex addict are no longer in play. You're willing to give up control, be in a state of not knowing, and make a space for your eroticism to emerge.

You value your partner as a novel and separate individual. You're as much concerned with your partner's sexual satisfaction as you are with your own. Each of you honors the other's erotic expression and, together, your unique erotic dance unfolds. Two dissolve into one, and a third energy of coupleship is birthed in a new way. You are no longer masculine or feminine in this dance; you meld into one entity and touch the silence of the universe.

Once it arrives, erotic sex cannot be chased or grasped at, for it shows itself when you're not looking. It can be quite ordinary as part of commonplace lovemaking or it can be raw and extraordinary. You'll know!

Patricia and Gary's Story

Two years into their recovery, Patricia and Gary have come a long way. In their late fifties, they've noticed that their biological sex drives aren't what they used to be. However, they have the maturity not to worry about this. Sometimes one of them is aroused and the other isn't, but that doesn't stop them from being sexual with each other. The good will is strong between them.

Patricia and Gary used the Four Cornerstones of Intimacy—self-knowledge, comfort and connection, responsibility with discernment, and empathy with emotion—to negotiate this level of trust. Over the years, they devoted themselves to only having sex when they knew they were present and available to themselves and one another. They took responsibility for talking about who they were and what they wanted sexually, which created a deeper level of intimacy between them. They then put their desires into action. As time went on, they took greater sexual risks with each other and found themselves falling more deeply in love. Patricia began to trust in Gary's honesty for the first time.

Today, if Gary slides up to Patricia while she's sleeping, she may offer her body as an act of friendly love. Sometimes she stays in a half-awake state that requires no effort on her part, focuses on the sensations in her body, feels her love for Gary, and languishes in being taken. Other times she wakes up and faces Gary directly, connecting and giving him the full force of her eyes, love, and passion. Both of them find these surprise encounters erotic.

They feel connected because they've done their work. Without it, this same encounter could be dissociative, mechanical, or only serving one of the parties. Yet for Gary and Patricia, it allows them to keep their emotional connection with each other strong.

Ally and Dan's Story

At the other end of the spectrum, erotic, joyous sex can be wildly carnal and grow from genital lust, as Ally and Dan experienced. Like Patricia and Gary, Ally and Dan had struggled through recovery and done their homework. They agreed that they felt connected and more in love with each other today then they could have imagined possible.

One afternoon, while Dan was on top, propped up on his hands, thrusting, Ally focused on breathing deeply into her abdomen and pelvis, delighting in watching Dan watch her masturbate herself. Her orgasm was so intense that she was convulsing in laughter. She laughed so hard that she was gasping for air and crying. Dan wasn't sure exactly what had happened, but he fell onto her and joined her in a contagious laughter. When Ally was calmer, she explained to Dan that her orgasm had been so pleasurable, she could hardly stand it.

Larry's Story

Erotic sex can transform trauma into healing, as in Larry's case. Throughout his childhood, Larry's mother gave him enemas for every minor ailment he had. As a married heterosexual adult with children, he repeated his trauma by seeking anonymous homosexual experiences that included anal penetration. After sufficiently healing his childhood trauma in the growth stage of his recovery, he admitted to himself that he still found anal stimulation arousing.

Through therapy, Larry accepted this as part of who he was and what he liked sexually without feeling ashamed. Only then could he ask his wife if she would participate in anal stimulation. He had to think about the third cornerstone—responsibility with discernment— meaning he had to take responsibility for his sexual preference even though he knew it might set up a triggering event for his wife. As a result, he and his wife had erotic, nonshaming sex that included anal stimulation for him.

Although he was afraid of being rejected, Larry asked his wife to do something that he had only asked strangers or prostitutes to do in the past. He knew that if he didn't ask her, he would fantasize about someone else doing it for him. His big fear was asking her for anal stimulation with her fingers while he penetrated her, but was surprised and pleased to learn his request aroused her. By using the second cornerstone—comfort and connection—his wife was able to comfort her anxieties, listen to her partner, and challenge herself to grow sexually. She was happy to give to him in this way.

Madeline and Jim's Story

Madeline and Jim are a good example of sex being a powerful healing energy experience. When she was a young girl, Madeline's neighbor had molested her repeatedly. He also sodomized and threatened her. He would cry to make her feel guilty if she reported him, so she endured the molestation instead of reporting it to an adult.

As a teenager, Madeline drank lots of alcohol to dull the pain this created and became an alcoholic. By young adulthood, she was engaging in multiple sexual experiences, repeating her trauma in sexually addictive ways with one abusive man after another. Finally, she got into Alcoholics Anonymous and a few years later, Sex and Love Addicts Anonymous. After a long journey of 12-step recovery and intensive therapy, Madeline was finally ready for a relationship, and Jim entered her life.

Jim was a smart, upstanding guy who'd been through his share of dysfunctional relationships. When he met Madeline, this bright, intelligent woman excited him. They dated for one year and started talking about their plans for marriage and a family. Jim was hesistant to move forward because he believed Madeline's molestation history was impeding their sexual relationship. He had grown watchful about how to be with her, constantly taking her emotional temperature to see if she was okay.

To her credit, Madeline told him to be more assertive and ask for what he wanted sexually. Jim agreed to stop caretaking and admitted that tracking her moods made him feel responsible for her well-being. He was happy to hear her speak her truth, which allowed him to feel freer. Jim's challenge was to take responsibility for himself and what he wanted sexually.

At this juncture, their therapy focused on how sex could be a healing experience for Madeline. The closer she grew to Jim, the more resistant to being sexual she became, and she worried about shutting down. Her next assignment? To pay full, honest attention to her energy emotionally and physically during sex.

Eventually, Madeline was willing to address her anger at her molester in therapy. Because her repressed feelings were affecting her sex life with Jim, the two of them had to decide how to deal with her healing within this context. We discussed how she and Jim could pace themselves during sex by slowing down, allowing Madeline to stay connected to her bodily sensations. She talked with him during sex and maintained eye contact. He was committed to stopping if he became aware she was drifting away from the present moment.

The tension between them lessened over time. They continued to stay in conversation and stopped worrying about what the other was thinking and experiencing. As old feelings arose, Madeline had bouts of depression and reported feeling sick. When she cried during sex, Jim held her through the tears, allowing her to release the little girl's pent-up rage. Both of them felt their hearts blast open in closeness. They finally accepted that the crying was the sex they craved. They didn't need to go any further at that point because her crying elicited a depth between them.

The stage was set for Madeline and Jim to move into and beyond the darkness of her past. Madeline admitted to being afraid of going there and of what she might say to Jim. Could he hear the horrible things she never got to say as a child? Jim reminded her that, yes, he did want to be a part of her healing process. After they talked through a few incidents, the healing continued, and they had an erotic, loving, sexual experience afterward.

Ultimately, I believe we heal our sexuality with and through one another. *No therapist can take you to the depths of your sexual soul like your lover can.*

When you're brave enough to surrender and take responsibility for joining with your partner, you experience a depth of connection that far surpasses the chemical rush of any sexually addictive exploit. Erotic sex makes sex addiction look like child's play because it requires the maturity and responsibility for oneself and mutual caring for each other that only an adult can muster. Role-playing and fantasy have their place in healthy sex.

From erotic sex, you begin to invite spiritual energies by virtue of the connection you've made with your truth and with each other. You slowly strip away your judgments, then your clothing, and finally your pride. You remove the illusion of who you think you are, take off the mask of the false and social self, surrender the need to look good, and drop your ego and your ideas of what is proper. Shame is banished from the scene and deep love takes its place.

✓ Erotic Intelligence Checklist for Chapter 10

❏ Fantasy is healthy, especially now that you've both learned to trust yourselves and each other.

❏ In adult sexuality, pay attention to your current fantasies and discuss them with your partner, listening to his or hers without reaction or judgment. Monitor your fantasies for euphoric recall and disconnection. Be sure to return to the moment and your deep connection with your partner.

❏ Erotic sex requires the maturity and responsibility for oneself and mutual caring for each other that only adults can muster.

11

Spiritualizing Sex

Love is our true destiny.
We do not find the meaning of life
by ourselves alone—we find it with another.
The meaning of our life is a secret that
has to be revealed to us in love,
by the one we love.

—Thomas Merton (1915–1968)

People speak of spiritual sex as an act unto itself, to be experienced and cherished. Yet spiritualizing sex is actually a movement of energy—feeling and emotion—that rises within you and moves into your sexual physicality as an alive, tender, erotic, or passionate expression. Your bodies move without inhibition so all the energy can flow out of you and between the two of you. *You allow spiritual energy to express its dance through you.*

Sexuality can be a profound demonstration of your love, and especially your freedom, to express and bond. Spiritual sex, then, combines how you express your love with the intentions or blessings you bring to your partnership.

How do you accomplish that? You allow for sexual connections with each other that elicit sweet, caring, loving, tender, and other profound expressions of your union. So before you begin your lovemaking session, take time for ritual. Sit face-to-face, make eye contact, and breathe deeply. Listen to your inner voice and tell your partner the intention you want to set for this merging. You might say something like this: "My intention is that, together, we heal our sexual wounds this evening" or "I bless our sexual union knowing that spirit expresses itself in and through us."

To honor the flow of your yin and yang—your masculine and feminine sides, or the equal and opposite values of all your feeling states and energies—consider practicing the following:

- Allow both positive and negative mind experiences. Try to release the negative thoughts by sharing them with your partner or breathing through them and releasing them on your own.
- Be present and stay present by not judging whether your sexual experience is sweet and tender or wild and carnal. Say "yes" to all aspects of yourself that show up.
- Adore each other's bodies. Allow yourself to feel both your masculine and feminine sides, your giving and receiving sides.
- Allow uninhibited releases of joy and intense bursts of energy.
- Blend lust and love with your human and spiritual natures.
- Be respectful of your experience at all times.

Why Spiritualize Sex?

In spiritual sex, you and your partner continue to dance—to move rhythmically, cooperatively, and harmoniously—and to further understand the ability to receive. Receiving requires that you accept the love, energy, passion, fear, or reluctance of your partner. You surrender—submit, yield, or abandon—yourself entirely, merging in the union. When you open your hearts, ecstasy flows, and your sex life is enriched with wonder and curiosity. You're dedicated to the exploration of yourself through each other. People who have become differentiated can let go with abandon and merge with another without losing themselves. In the process of doing this, they touch the divine—and so can you.

When you spiritualize sex, you accept each other in partnership and use sexuality as a sacred means to fulfill and express yourselves. You lift yourselves into ecstasy and passion. Spiritual sex can give you the feeling that you're connecting to something larger than yourself or your partner. Together, you merge into a union that has no reference to self or other. Through the spiritual sexual act, you can experience consciousness meeting consciousness—an unbounded wholeness that's no longer personal—and yet is *deeply* personal because you touch the heavens through your partner. In this sacred space, you celebrate that you are spiritual beings sharing your human experiences.

Spiritualizing sex takes willingness to create a spiritual bond through a commitment to completely know yourself with your partner. You willingly and eagerly grow with another person and surrender to the relationship. You allow for differences to be handled mutually. You hold the intention to always return to unity or harmony. When you relate to each other from the heart and soul, your essence is kind, honest, and compassionate. You see beyond personalities, without projections and idealizations. You see life through your *god eyes*.

At this stage, something new happens: You are able to tolerate self-ish desire for pleasure and not take your partner's selfish desires personally. You are both centered and, paradoxically, able to lose yourselves to each other and touch the divine. You honor the spirit within and recognize your partner as a manifestation of the spirit. For each of you, sex becomes a merging encounter, two streams flowing together, a blend of God's creation.

Sensual, Spiritual Experience

Spiritualized sex is a sensual experience that gives rise to passion and a deepening that takes you beyond your personality to a place of unity and wholeness. In the moment, everything you've learned about holding the tension of nervous excitement is still true. Be careful not to disappear on yourself or your partner by disconnecting or dissociating. Instead, become aware of the energy when the tingles you feel deepen to sensual pleasures. Let your passion rise and spiral into ecstasy.

This can be likened to a spiritual experience while sitting in meditation. Finding a comfortable place to sit, you become ever so still, noticing your thoughts and keeping your attention on your breathing. As soon as you do, the tension of every ache, cramp, and pain surfaces and screams for attention. Being aware, you acknowledge the tension and allow the pain, ache, and fear to coalesce into a swirling energy that rises and bursts out of your head like an orgasm. Then, you sit in silence—no thoughts, only breathing and a freeing feeling of expanded consciousness.

How to Spiritualize Sex

In his book *Blue Truth*, David Deida states, "The masculine directs, the feminine invites."[1] To be true to the nature of your gender, the feminine opens to energy and invites the masculine in. The masculine directs the energy to empower the feminine to feel it, be warmed by it, glow in it. The energy spreads through the feminine and moves right back to the masculine, then with purpose moves with the feminine—rocking, holding, thrusting, or releasing.

When you play these inviting and directing roles with each other, mutual trust and understanding develop. This trust allows for your explorations within the sexual experience. You focus, tense, feel, relax, and open up to each other.

Especially focus on directing your energy through actions like gazing into your partner's eyes and tracing circles on his or her back. Whatever titillating experiences you create, do so with full attention. Feel the touch, softness, or penetration fully, then open further through breathing, eye contact, or relaxation.

During sex, stop, relax, and notice the sexual excitement in your bodies. Breathe together and feel the warmth as it radiates throughout. Notice what you feel in this engagement. Does time stop? Do you notice that your thoughts are quiet? You are in an ecstatic meditation with your lover, with no pressure or expectation. This can be your spiritual path.

Rituals Set the Stage

Rituals prepare each of you to meet the sacred in each other. Breathing, prayer, or meditation sets the stage for inviting your highest selves to a sexual feast. See what happens when the feminine worships the masculine and the masculine serves the feminine.

Couples in therapy ask me why ritual is important, yet everyone understands why children benefit from the ritual of a shared dinner and conversation that centers on their lives. Like two martial artists bowing to each other in greeting, ritual can enhance your sex life.

Rituals start as simple acts of preparation or kindness, such as lighting a candle. Repeated rituals train your body and mind to focus fully on the event and engage your partner with heart and respect. In effect, rituals create the time, space, and energy to connect with each other.

Just as we come to love the holidays every year or enjoy annual birthday celebrations, we look forward to rituals because they're comfortable interludes when we feel safe and can be completely genuine.

Important Rituals for Connection

Consider these rituals that support your partnership's connection and empathy:

- Set up your physical space together with the intention to convert the sexual act into a meditative, spiritual experience.
- Exchange small gifts with your partner based on what you know about him or her.
- State a vow in which you recognize and honor that you are responsible for how you have changed your lives and partnership.

To extend the pre-orgasm experience:

- Be sexual with your clothes on. Kiss, fondle, and arouse by touching through or under your clothes. Let the arousal reach a peak without orgasm. If either person feels close to orgasm, ask your partner to stop. After each person reaches this pre-orgasmic peak, take a breather to build the energy again. When you converse, remember to talk in the present tense to keep you present with each other.

- Breathe together, ideally using Full-Wave Breathing, as described below. Stretch out on your bed, side by side, facing each other. Hug each other and breathe in opposite rhythms. When one person breathes in, the other exhales, and vice versa. Continue sharing your breaths until you are fully relaxed.

- Find the most sensitive part of your partner's body without being told. Pay attention to cues such as moaning or writhing, but don't talk. Signs that a woman is aroused include changes in breathing, skin flushing, aroused nipples, and vaginal lubrication. Besides an erection, signs indicating a male is aroused include erect nipples, changes in breathing patterns, writhing, and fluid at the tip of the penis.

Breathing to Focus, Open, Relax

Spiritualizing sex requires being in touch with your breathing in a deep way. The International Breath Institute (www.international breathinstitute.com) teaches Full-Wave Breathing for purposes of relaxing and opening the body, focusing your energy or intention, and reenergizing the body and mind. You can use Full-Wave Breathing when preparing for sex as part of any ritual. It's a three-step process—not a one-breath event, but a conscious, circular experience. The inhale and exhale seem separate at first, yet the more you relax and focus on the breathing, your breath becomes a continuous flow, and sensations heighten while tensions release. You are fully present with your partner.

Here is a description of the three steps in Full-Wave Breathing that help you consciously control your breath so you can control your responses in all situations.

Step 1

Breathe into the abdomen, relaxing and opening the lower half of your body. Most people hold their breath during orgasm and tense up from poor breathing habits.

With your partner or by yourself, expand your belly as you inhale slowly and comfortably. Make your exhale quick, not prolonged, as your abdomen deflates and relaxes. Do this first step for five, ten, or even fifty breath cycles to raise the sexual energy.

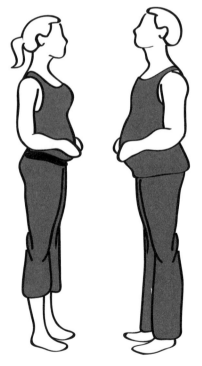

Breathing as suggested provides the additional benefits of lowering blood pressure and cholesterol. People also use the abdominal breath for toning muscles and relaxing tension from indigestion.

Figure 11.1. Abdominal Breathing

Step 2

Increase the breath wave into the diaphragm area by continuing to expand the rib cage and solar plexus. While inhaling, mentally count "one" and expand the abdomen, then count "two" and expand the diaphragm. Exhale normally without prolonging it to let the abdomen and diaphragm relax. By placing your palms on the lower rib cages, you'll feel the expansion and deflation.

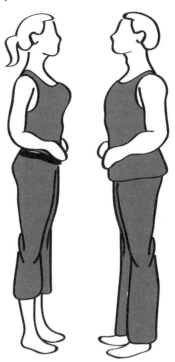

Figure 11.2. Expand Your Breathing

Step 3

Expand the breath wave into the chest on the mental count of "three." While inhaling, silently count "one" and expand the abdomen; count "two" and expand the diaphragm; without pause, count "three" and pull up or expand the air into your chest. Then exhale as a short sigh, relax, and repeat at least ten times, if not more. The more repetition, the brighter and lighter you will feel.

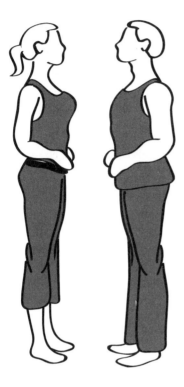

Figure 11.3. Full-Wave Breathing

If you've never retrained your breathing patterns for focus, relaxation, and vitality, then you'll need practice time to allow the flow of your breath to become easy, natural, and fluid. Breathing a full wave with each other brings alignment and openness as a couple. You'll find that your expanded breathing can carry you to heights of sensation and depths of loving feelings as it modulates your hearts' rhythms.

Use Full-Wave Breathing to connect and align, and then expand your rituals and preparation for spiritualizing sex.

Creating the Sacred Space

Breathing and meditation are tools available to help you create a peaceful, sacred state within you. Just as it's important to prepare your bodily environments for the sacred intention of spiritual sex, preparing your space depends on your preferences and your partner's requests. Throughout your recovery, you've been encouraged to take risks, knowing that your fears will arise. Trusting your partner and the solidity of your relationship is key to facing these challenges.

To create your sacred space, take an ordinary room and turn it into a sanctuary, transforming it from the mundane into a space of trust and safety that lets you venture into the unknown. Consider taking these steps to eliminate distractions and add a peaceful ambience:

- Dress in sensual, comfortable clothing.
- Clear clutter from the space.
- Dim the lights, use candles, light the fireplace.
- Turn off the television and computer, cover the clocks, and put any phones in another room. Even cover the television and computer with a beautiful piece of fabric.
- Prepare fresh linens, comfortable robes, soft comforters—whatever adds to your comfort and pleasure.
- Add small luxuries and thoughtful touches: music, aromatherapy, a small fountain with trickling water, flowers, incense, or foods such as fruits, nuts, or sweets.

Think of Sex as Prayer

Think about sex as prayer. Think about sex as life affirming. Think about sex as rejuvenation, as being inspired to go out in the world knowing you're loved. Appealing and creative, spiritual sexual energy builds confidence and makes you feel whole.

When I think about sex as a prayer, I visualize the Tantric practice of sitting together with a man's penis inserted into the woman's vagina while in the cross-legged position. Tantra literally means "loom, thread, web, ritual, or doctrine." It's a religion that formed approximately 1,000 BC and attributes everything sexual to the feminine. Tantra is "the positive Indian teaching concerning the physical manifestations of sex."[2] The traditional depiction is of the woman sitting on the man's lap with their heads touching. The sense of breathing and communing with each other engenders the image of creating a flow of energy together. The idea is to sit without thrusting, noticing the subtle changes of warming sensuality in your bodies.

As your feelings rise in this position, trust your intuition to inform you of your prayer. You may find yourself overwhelmed with gratitude for your life, amazed at the miracle you are, and thankful that you put in the time and energy to heal yourself and your relationship.

Your prayer may come as a feeling of deep inner peace, or it may feel like a sense of freedom in the form of abandon with each other. Trust what comes through you and let it be. Relish your feeling and share your thoughts with your partner.

Feelings and Forms of Sex

Spiritual sex reflects the attitude of respect and actions of kindness. It can also be fun and reverential, giving you the freedom to try things your way, not in prescribed ways learned in our families and our cultures.

Sex in its most elevated state can take different forms. When you've been having connected sex, taking time to have slow, erotic orgasms or a spontaneous quickie can both be fun because they allow you to reach a deeper genuineness. After all, the spontaneous moments are part of what people do when they have busy lives, jobs, and children.

When loving qualities and the Four Cornerstones of Intimacy become tangible parts of your relationship, short sexual interludes

Greg and Colleen's Story

Greg's mother died when he was five years old and his sisters were eight and ten. Shortly after her death, his father married a woman who already had two small children. Feeling harried caring for five children, she didn't pay much attention to Greg. He grew up seeking female attention and quickly learned that sex was a way to get the touch and consideration he desperately needed. But once he got married, he was unable to break his addictive sexual patterns. It wasn't until Greg and his wife, Colleen, were four years into their recovery that he could ask for what he needed without judgment and shame silencing him.

Sex addicts often can't tolerate closeness for several reasons: their nervous systems aren't used to it, they don't feel entitled to it because of shame, or it feels too dangerously vulnerable. Greg's reclaiming his sexuality involved learning what he needed and how to tolerate the intensity of his feelings once he got it. Part of setting his intention to heal was asking Colleen to hold him like a five-year-old. He begged to be cuddled, stroked, held, and told that he was loved.

She willingly took on this role, which forced her to tolerate the discomfort that the feeling of being motherly with him brought up for her. This motherly role was distinctly different from the one she'd played during the years when Greg was acting out. It was as if she had a child who wasn't accountable for his life on her hands.

But she didn't collapse into resentment and judgment of Greg. Instead, she was able to hold on to her identity as a wife and lover who was giving and nurturing to her partner. This allowed Greg to

> reveal his most vulnerable self to her. Together, they created an intimacy born out of knowing each other deeply. This intimacy allowed them to heal both individually and as a couple. Tenderness on both of their parts opened their hearts and led them to having deeper, more connected sex.

bring a different expression to your great relationship. The idea—always—is to stay connected and create spiritual foundations in many actions throughout your day, with sex being one of them.

Whether you're having a pillow fight or chasing each other around the house, that sense of rough-and-tumble play can lead to joyous giggling and fun sex that turns passionate and erotic when your bodies heat up. You're responding to each other. Sex doesn't have to be serious. Having a playful attitude takes you past any notion of getting it right or any sense of self-importance. Quarrels can be easily neutralized with laughter and playfulness.

Healing Through Spiritual Sex

The deep healing that takes place through spiritual sex can never happen in a therapy session. In sex, there's you and your partner and the resonance between you. Next comes the meaning you create out of what arises reflected by what you're feeling. Phenomenal healing can take place in spiritual sexuality; in a gaze, pose, or special position, the union of two becomes one, your healing embodied.

Much healing can occur through the sexual act with a person you love and trust if the two of you can stay with each other during your most vulnerable moments. You enter into a sacred space, this unknown territory, from which you'll emerge into new and unexpected states of being.

Are you willing to step into the unknown? Are you willing to say that this is your prayer together as a couple for meaning-making, for affirming life? If so, then you can explore universes that no therapist could ever prescribe or recommend. The gratification that comes from such healing is more extraordinary than anything you've ever known before.

Dr. M. Scott Peck, author of *The Road Less Traveled,* observed that those lost in the compulsive, driven pursuit of sex are actually searching for spirituality.[3] I agree that sex addicts are looking for a transcendent experience within their trauma. Yes, they're looking for it in the right place through sex, but they're looking for it in the wrong way. When sex is disconnected from spirit, then misery, emptiness, and depression inevitably set in.

Great spiritual teachers throughout the ages have stated that orgasm is the closest some people come to a spiritual experience because of the momentary loss of self. Why is this true? Because with spiritual sex, you move beyond orgasm into a connection with yourself, your partner, and the divine—recognizing them all as one. You can now approach spiritual sex fully because you have healed from the shame of addiction. Through recovery, you recognize yourself as a manifestation of something good rather than something shameful or bad. As all shame is erased, you feel desirable—with your sexual desire coming from a sense of internal fullness. You no longer seek to assuage your feelings of emptiness with meaningless sexual acts devoid of a soul connection.

Sexuality and spirituality become linked because you have decided what they mean to you. Indeed, you can no longer talk about or include one without the other. You bring your spirit—the highest manifestation of your potential—into sex so you can connect deeply with the one you love.

We rarely get messages like these from our families and culture. Despite centuries of literature that testifies to the power and beauty of sex, rarely is sexual energy equated with self-love, laughter, spontaneity, and spirituality. And yet, if sex were a meaningless act, much of the shame and obsession around it would not exist.

Thomas Moore, author of *The Soul of Sex: Cultivating Life as an Act of Love,* reminds us that Eros as defined by the Greeks is a lofty and spiritual kind of love. He writes, "Sex keeps us connected to our deepest natures and links us to our roots. In that way it expands the source from which we live our lives."[4]

Greek literature refers to love as the force that holds the universe together, and human love is one small form of this greater love. Moore suggests that we reinstate Eros as a sense of holiness in our day-to-day activities and in the nature of all things. This would elevate our reductionist view of sex from something dirty, small, and irrelevant to a force in all of us and in all things powerful, vital, and strong.

Continue to Explore Your Sexuality

Don't let yourself be daunted by this process of sexual growth and deepening. You'll experience both peaks and valleys as you continue your sexual exploration, just as you did in early recovery. When you were slogging through the valleys of your early recovery, you thought you'd never see your way out. But through perseverance and your desire to be a better person, you did.

Today, you have a new source from which to live your life—your sexual vitality. Envision this newfound vitality as the next stage of moving into the best sexual health you've ever had. As always, you can take it one step at a time. Remember to use the tools that make you feel good about yourself, that increase intimacy and excitement. You've arrived at a new vista, and the view is clearer than when you set out on this journey. You have more knowledge, confidence, and experience with your partner than you've ever had before—and that makes you more erotically intelligent.

Possessing erotic intelligence, you now have the ability to make sexual choices that affirm life in healthy, imaginative, and exciting ways. One of the great challenges of living a recovered life is to experience this kind of sex with a partner with whom you feel safe, secure, and connected while revealing the depths of your erotic, sexual self. You've come this far. You have what it takes.

✓ Erotic Intelligence Checklist for Chapter 11

❏ Rituals prepare each partner to meet the sacred in each other. Breathing, prayer, and/or meditation can set the stage for inviting your highest selves to a sexual feast.

❏ Full-Wave Breathing helps you relax and open your body, focus your energy or intention, and reenergize your body and mind. It provides an excellent preamble to spiritual sex.

❏ Spiritual sex suggests that you move beyond orgasm into the connection with yourself, your partner, and the divine, recognizing them all as one.

Afterword

In active addiction, sex addicts are in relationship with sex, not with people. Recovery involves creating a relationship with yourself first and foremost, then with others, and finally with one significant other.

As human beings, we naturally seek attachment in order to grow, learn, and experience life. Without this kind of contact with others, we live in isolation, and eventually our brains, bodies, and souls wither and die. Our sexuality is a vital energy that's part of this alive state in our bodies. Sexually expressing that state is the ultimate representation of our love for ourselves and for another. However, when they're abused, sex and sexual energy can become weapons to be used against ourselves and others. As a culture, when our shame has us distorting the good and the beautiful in sex, it's no wonder that violence in pornography increases constantly.

Healing our sexuality means we heal the core of who we are individually and collectively. Why? So we can forgive ourselves and others who may have hurt us. The "preparation" referred to in the Rilke quotation above includes the work it takes to get clarity about where we've come from, who we are, and what we want in our lives. Once that process is under way, only then can we join with another person who will enrich our personal growth and development.

Now is the time to risk exploring, knowing, and revealing yourself as a sexual being to another person—especially to your partner. Once you take the leap to finally lay bare and heal your sexuality, you're on the road to change. As Mohandas Gandhi said, "You must be the change you wish to see in the world."

Above all, consider this: *The greatest gift we can give ourselves, our children, and our world is to live well and love well.*

May you love well!

Resources for Support

National Therapy Resources

Sexual Addiction Resources/Dr. Patrick Carnes

www.sexhelp.com

An online resource developed by Dr. Patrick Carnes that offers books, exercises, and referrals from a leader in this field.

Society for the Advancement of Sexual Health (SASH)

www.sash.net

Telephone: (706) 356-7031

E-mail: sash@sash.net

Formerly known as the National Council for Sexual Addiction and Compulsivity, SASH serves both treatment professionals and recovering individuals. It provides resources and information on addiction therapists, treatment centers, and support groups.

American Association of Sexuality Educators, Counselors, and Therapists (AASECT)

www.aasect.org

Telephone: (804) 752-0026

E-mail: aasect@aasect.org

A not-for-profit, interdisciplinary professional organization made up of individuals who share an interest in promoting understanding of human sexuality and healthy sexual behavior. It provides resources and information on sex therapy and how to locate a sex therapist.

American Association for Marriage and Family Therapy (AAMFT)

www.aamft.org

Telephone: (703) 838-9808

The professional association for the field of marriage and family therapy representing the professional interests of more than 24,000 marriage and family therapists throughout the United States, Canada, and abroad. The AAMFT is involved with the problems, needs, and changing patterns of couples and family relationships. It provides resources and information on couples and families, and how to locate a marriage/family therapist.

Center for Healthy Sex (CHS)

www.thecenterforhealthysex.com

Telephone: (310) 335-0997

E-mail: info@thecenterforhealthysex.com

Under the direction of the author, this outpatient treatment center in Southern California specializes in providing treatment for issues related to sexual addiction and sexuality. CHS offers an intensive outpatient program (IOP) for local and national clients. Other services include individual, group, and couple therapy, workshops, and continuing education courses for therapy professionals. Visit the website for more information, articles, and resources.

International Breath Institute

http://internationalbreathinstitute.com

Telephone: (817) 847-8216

E-mail: thomasgoode@earthlink.net

The International Breath Institute teaches people the keys to wellness in body, mind, and spirit through Full-Wave Breathing and its awareness-expanding programs. Methods are safe, natural, simple to use, self-empowering, and easy to perform.

International Institute for Trauma and Addiction Professionals (IITAP)

www.iitap.com

Telephone: (480) 575-6853

E-mail: info@iitap.com

The certified sex addiction therapist (CSAT) designation is offered by the International Institute for Trauma and Addiction Professionals (IITAP). The CSAT certification provides formal training and knowledge in the task-centered approach for the treatment of sexual addiction and sexual compulsivity.

12-Step Programs for Couples

Recovering Couples Anonymous (RCA)

www.recovering-couples.org

Telephone: (718) 794-1456; Toll Free for United States and Canada 1-877-663-2317

E-mail: wso-rca@recovering-couples.org

This 12-step program is national in scope and focuses on recovery issues experienced by couples affected by sex addiction. Both partners (addict and co-addict) are encouraged to attend. All committed couples are welcome.

12-Step Programs for Sex Addicts

Sex Addicts Anonymous (SAA)

www.sexaa.org

National: (800) 477-8191

E-mail: info@saa-recovery.org

A 12-step program for sex addicts and some offenders, SAA offers a good mix of gay- and straight-oriented meetings. Women attend some meetings.

Sexual Compulsives Anonymous (SCA)

www.sca-recovery.org

National: (800) 977-4325 (977-HEAL)

A 12-step program designed primarily for sex addicts, SCA is concentrated mostly in major urban areas. Its meetings often reflect a sizable gay presence. Women attend some meetings.

Sex and Love Addicts Anonymous (SLAA)

www.slaafws.org

National: (781) 255-8825

A 12-step program designed for sex addicts and individuals with patterns of unhealthy romantic relationships, SLAA has a greater female presence than many other recovery programs. Some meetings are for women only.

Sexaholics Anonymous (SA)

www.sa.org

National: (866) 424-8777

E-mail: saico@sa.org

A 12-step program for sex addicts and sex offenders. Most meetings are composed of men. The least gay-supportive of the 12-step recovery programs for sex addiction, SA bases its definition of sobriety on traditional concepts of marriage. However, individual groups vary in their degree of openness to gay, lesbian, bisexual, and transgender (GLBT) issues.

Sexual Recovery Anonymous (SRA)

www.sexualrecovery.org

24-hour Hotline: (212) 340-4650

E-mail: info@sexualrecovery.org

A 12-step program similar to SA except the phrase "committed relationship" is used instead of "marriage." Meetings are limited in number but open to everyone in sexual recovery. Regional contact numbers for groups in the United States and abroad are available at SRA's website.

12-Step Programs for Significant Others

S-Anon International

www.sanon.org

National: (800) 210-8141 or (615) 833-3152

E-mail: sanon@sanon.org

A companion program to SA, S-Anon is a 12-step program for spouses/partners of sex addicts and sex offenders. Most meetings are primarily made up of married women.

Codependents of Sex Addicts (COSA)

www.cosa-recovery.org

National: (763) 537-6904

E-mail: info@cosa-recovery.org

A companion program to SAA, COSA is a 12-step program for partners and significant others of sex addicts and sex offenders. Both men and women attend groups.

Codependents of Sex and Love Addicts Anonymous (COSLAA)

www.coslaa.org

Help Line: (860) 456-0032

A 12-step support group for the recovery of family, friends, and significant others whose lives have been affected by their relationship with someone addicted to sex and love. COSLAA, also known as CoSex and Love Addicts Anonymous, reaches out to the suffering individuals eighteen years or older, regardless of sexual orientation, gender, or relationship status.

Additional Resources

Erotic Intelligence has been written to assist you in moving toward a healthy sex life through writing exercises and suggestions. The exercises invite you to examine your deepest fears, insecurities, and blocks around your sexuality. Because restoring sexuality after recovery from sexual addiction is often a difficult, challenging, and painful process, you may find you need a qualified therapist to assist you. How do you find the right one?

I recommend going to the Society for the Advancement of Sexual Health website, www.sash.net, which features a therapist directory. There you will find therapists devoted to the treatment of sexual addiction. For a higher level of expertise, look for therapists who are certified sex addiction therapists (CSATs). After their names, you'll see the designation CSAT as well as the type of license they hold. To find a certified sex therapist, go to the website for the American Association of Sex Educators, Counselors, and Therapists, www.aasect.org, which also features a therapist directory.

I also recommend the Center for Healthy Sex (CHS). Since 2005, CHS has offered extensive treatment of sexual addiction for individuals, their partners, and couples. Its intensive outpatient program

(IOP) is a comprehensive two-week program that assists people in becoming sexually sober and in moving toward their own erotic intelligence. This is especially helpful for those who cannot maintain sexual sobriety in an outpatient setting or who cannot afford an inpatient hospital stay. Using cutting-edge protocols, CHS tailors each individual's program to his/her specific needs. CHS also conducts programs for therapists and the general public, including a monthly continuing education lecture series, weekend workshops, and national lectures.

For speaking engagements for your organization on erotic intelligence or any topics related to sexual addiction, contact:

Center for Healthy Sex
9911 W. Pico Boulevard, Suite 700
Los Angeles, CA 90035
Phone: (310) 335-0997
E-mail: info@thecenterforhealthysex.com
Website: www.thecenterforhealthysex.com
Blog site: www.sexaddictionlosangeles.com

Notes

Chapter 1

1   A. N. Schore, *Affect Regulation and the Repair of the Self* (New York: W. W. Norton, 2003), 12–13.

2   M. F. Soloman, *Lean on Me: The Power of Positive Dependency in Intimate Relationships* (New York: Kensington, 2004), 183.

3   R. Grigg, *The Tao of Relationships: A Balancing of Man and Woman* (New York: Bantam Books, 1989), 89.

4   M. E. Kerr and M. Bowen, *Family Evaluation: An Approach Based on Bowen Theory* (New York: W. W. Norton, 1978), 63.

Chapter 2

1   A. Goodman, "Neurobiology of addiction: An integrative review," *Biochemical Pharmacology* 75 (2008): 266–322.

2   N. Dodgie, *The Brain that Changes Itself: Stories of Personal Triumph from the Frontiers of Brain Science* (New York: Penguin Books, 2007), 106.

Chapter 3

1   A. Bartels and S. Zeki, "The neural basis of romantic love," *NeuroReport* 11, 17 (2000): 3829–34.

2   H. E. Fisher, *Why We Love: The Nature and Chemistry of Romantic Love* (New York: Henry Holt, 2004), 78.

3   Aviva Patz, "Will your marriage last?" *Psychology Today* Vol. 33 No. 1 (Jan/Feb 2000): 58

4   J. Abrahms Spring and M. Spring, *After the Affair: Healing the Pain and Rebuilding Trust After a Partner Has Been Unfaithful* (New York: HarperPaperbacks, 1996), 247–48.

5   L. J. Pitkow, C. A. Sharer, X. Ren, T. R. Insel, E. F. Terwilliger, and L. J. Young, "Facilitation of affiliation and pair-bond formation by vasopressin receptor gene transfer into the ventral forebrain of a monogamous vole," *Journal of Neuroscience* 21, 18 (2001): 7392–96.

6   L. E. Shapiro and D. A. Dewsbury, "Differences in affiliative behavior, pair bonding, and vaginal cytology in two species of vole (*Microtus ochrogaster* and *M. montanus*)," *Journal of Comparative Psychology* 104, 3 (1990): 268–74.

7   H. E. Fisher, *Why We Love: The Nature and Chemistry of Romantic Love* (New York: Henry Holt, 2004), 110–12.

8   Ibid., 113–16.

Chapter 4

1   E. T. Robinson, *Why Aren't You More Like Me? Styles and Skills for Leading and Living with Credibility*, 2nd ed. (Sumas, WA: Consulting Resource Group International, 1994).

2   J. Y. W. Cheng and E. M. L. Ng, "Body mass index, physical activity and erectile dysfunction: A U-shaped relationship from population-based study," *International Journal of Obesity* 13 (2007): 1571–78.

3   L. D. Hamilton, E. A. Fogle, and C. M. Meston, "The roles of testosterone and alpha-amylase in exercise-induced sexual arousal in women," *Journal of Sexual Medicine* 5 (2008): 845–53.

4   M. Castleman, *Great Sex: A Man's Guide to the Secret Principles of Total-Body Sex* (Emmaus, PA: Rodale Press, 2004), 54.

Chapter 5

1   S. Carnes, ed., *Mending a Shattered Heart: A Guide for Partners of Sex Addicts* (Carefree, AZ: Gentle Path Press, 2008), 54.

Chapter 7

1 P. C. Whybrow, *American Mania: When More Is Not Enough* (New York: W. W. Norton, 2006), 92–96.

2 W. Maltz and L. Maltz, *The Porn Trap: The Essential Guide to Overcoming Problems Caused by Pornography* (New York: HarperCollins, 2008), 23.

3 M. L. Chivers and J. M. Bailey, "A sex difference in features that elicit genital response," *Biological Psychology* 70, 2 (2008): 115–20.

4 Ibid.

5 B. R. Komisaruk, C. Beyer-Flores, and B. Whipple, *The Science of Orgasm* (Baltimore, MD: Johns Hopkins University Press, 2006), 73, 200–207.

Chapter 8

1 B. B. Barratt, *Ten Keys to Successful Sexual Partnering* (Bloomington, IN: Xlibris, 2005), 39.

Chapter 9

1 M. Lüscher, *The Colors of Love: Getting to Know Your Romantic Self Through Color* (New York: St. Martin's Press, 1996), 9.

2 M. Castleman, *Great Sex: A Man's Guide to the Secret Principles of Total-Body Sex* (Emmaus, PA: Rodale Press, 2004), 15.

3 R. J. Levin, "Vocalised sounds and human sex," *Sexual and Relationship Therapy* 21, 1 (2006): 99–107.

4 N. L. McCoy and L. Pitino, "Pheromonal influences on sociosexual behavior in young women," *Physiology and Behavior* 75, 3 (2002): 367–75.

5 Office of Health Education, University of Pennsylvania, http://www.vpul.upenn.edu/ohe/library/Sexhealth/articles/Aphrodisiacs.htm.

Chapter 10

1 B. W. McCarthy and E. McCarthy, *Discovering Your Couple Sexual Style* (Routledge: New York and London, 2009), 59.

Chapter 11

1 D. Deida, *Blue Truth* (Boulder, CO: Sounds True, 2005), 117.

2 J. Mumford, *Ecstasy Through Tantra* (St. Paul, MN: Llewellyn, 1993), 18, 20.

3 M.Scott Peck, *Further Along the Road Less Traveled* (New York: Simon & Schuster, 1993), 226–229.

4 T. Moore, *The Soul of Sex: Cultivating Life as an Act of Love* (New York: HarperCollins, 1998), 17.

Bibliography

Adams, K., and M. Alexandre. *When He's Married to Mom: How to Help Mother-Enmeshed Men Open Their Hearts to True Love and Commitment.* New York: Fireside, 2007.

Alcoholics Anonymous: The Story of How Many Thousands of Men and Women Have Recovered from Alcoholism. 4th ed. New York: Alcoholics Anonymous World Services, 2002.

Anand, M. *The Art of Sexual Ecstasy: The Path of Sacred Sexuality for Western Lovers.* New York: Jeremy P. Tarcher/Putnam, 1989.

Bader, M. J. *Arousal: The Secret Logic of Sexual Fantasies.* New York: St. Martin's Press. 2002.

Barratt, B. B. *Ten Keys to Successful Sexual Partnering.* Bloomington, IN: Xlibris Corporation, 2005.

Brizendine, L. *The Female Brain.* New York: Broadway Books, 2006.

Carnes, P. *Don't Call It Love: Recovery from Sexual Addiction.* New York: Bantam Books, 1991.

———. *Facing the Shadow: Starting Sexual and Relationship Recovery.* Carefree, AZ: Gentle Path Press, 2001.

———. *Out of the Shadows: Understanding Sexual Addiction.* Center City, MN: Hazelden, 1983.

Carnes, S., ed. *Mending a Shattered Heart: A Guide for Partners of Sex Addicts.* Carefree, AZ: Gentle Path Press, 2008.

245

Castleman, M. *Great Sex: A Man's Guide to the Secret Principles of Total-Body Sex.* Emmaus, PA: Rodale, 2004.

Chia, Mantak, Maneewan Chia, D. Abrams, and R. Carlton-Abrams. *The Multi-Orgasmic Couple: Sexual Secrets Every Couple Should Know.* New York: HarperCollins, 2000.

Deida, D. *The Enlightened Sex Manual: Sexual Skills for the Superior Lover.* Boulder, CO: Sounds True, 2004.

Doidge, N. *The Brain that Changes Itself: Stories of Personal Triumph from the Frontiers of Brain Science.* New York: Penguin, 2007.

Fisher, H. E. *Why We Love: The Nature and Chemistry of Romantic Love.* New York: Henry Holt, 2004.

Gibran, K. *The Prophet.* New York: Alfred A. Knopf, 1997.

Goodman, V. "Neurobiology of addiction: An integrative review." *Biochemical Pharmacology* 75 (2007): 266–322.

Grigg, R. *The Tao of Relationships: A Guide to Love and Friendship for a New Age.* New York: Bantam Doubleday Dell, 1989.

Kasl, C. S. *If the Buddha Dated: A Handbook for Finding Love on a Spiritual Path.* New York: Penguin/Arkana, 1999.

Katehakis, A. "Affective neuroscience and the treatment of sexual addiction." *Journal of Sexual Addiction and Compulsivity,* 16 (2009): 1–31.

Katherine, A. *Boundaries: Where You End and I Begin.* New York: Fireside/Parkside, 1991.

Kerr, M. E., and M. Bowen. *Family Evaluation: An Approach Based on Bowen Theory.* New York: W. W. Norton, 1978.

Komisaruk, B. R., C. Beyer-Flores, and B. Whipple. *The Science of Orgasm.* Baltimore, MD: Johns Hopkins University Press, 2006.

Lewis, T., F. Amini, and R. Lannon. *A General Theory of Love.* New York: Random House, 2000.

Maltz, W., and L. Maltz. *The Porn Trap: The Essential Guide to Overcoming Problems Caused by Pornography.* New York: HarperCollins, 2008.

McCarthy, B. W., and M. E. Metz. *Men's Sexual Health: Fitness for Satisfying Sex.* New York: Routledge Taylor & Francis, 2008.

McDaniel, K. *Ready to Heal: Women Facing Love, Sex, and Relationship Addiction.* Gentle Path Press, 2008.

Merton, T. *Disputed Questions*. New York: Farrar, Straus and Giroux, 1977.

————. *Love and Living*. New York: Harcourt Brace, 1985.

————. *Mystics and Zen Masters*. New York: Farrar, Straus and Giroux, 1987.

Moore, T. *Care of the Soul: A Guide for Cultivating Depth and Sacredness in Everyday Life*. New York: HarperCollins, 1992.

————. *The Soul of Sex: Cultivating Life as an Act of Love*. New York: HarperCollins, 1998.

Mumford, J. *Ecstasy Through Tantra*. St. Paul, MN: Llewellyn, 1993.

Odier, D. *Desire: The Tantric Path to Awakening*. Rochester, VT: Inner Traditions International, 2001.

Panksepp, J. *Affective Neuroscience: The Foundations of Human and Animal Emotions*. New York: Oxford Press, 1998.

Peck, M. Scott. *Further Along the Road Less Traveled*. New York: Simon & Schuster, 1993.

Schnarch, D. M. *Constructing the Sexual Crucible: An Integration of Sexual and Marital Therapy*. New York: W. W. Norton, 1991.

————. *Intimacy and Desire: Awaken the Passion in Your Relationship*. New York: Beaufort Press, 2009.

Schore, A. N. *Affect Regulation and the Origin of the Self: The Neurobiology of Emotional Development*. Hillsdale, NJ: Lawrence Erlbaum Associates, 1994.

————. *Affect Regulation and the Repair of the Self*. New York: W. W. Norton, 2003.

Siegel, D. J. *The Developing Mind: How Relationships and the Brain Interact to Shape Who We Are*. New York: Guilford Press, 1999.

Solomon, M. F. *Lean on Me: The Power of Positive Dependency in Intimate Relationships*. New York: Kensington, 1994.

————. *Narcissism and Intimacy: Love and Marriage in an Age of Confusion*. New York: W. W. Norton, 1989.

Solomon, M. F., and S. Tatkin. *Love and War in Intimate Relationships: A Psychobiological Approach to Couple Therapy*. New York: W. W. Norton, 2009.

Spring, Janis Abrahms, with Michael Spring. *After the Affair: Healing the Pain and Rebuilding Trust When a Partner Has Been Unfaithful*. New York: HarperCollins, 1996.

Sudo, P. T. *Zen Sex: The Way of Making Love*. New York: HarperCollins, 2000.

Taylor, K. *Life's Too Short for Tantric Sex: 50 Shortcuts to Sexual Ecstasy.* Lewes East Sussex, UK: Ivy Press Ltd., 2003.

Tiefer, L. *Sex Is Not a Natural Act and Other Essays.* Boulder, CO: Westview Press, 1995.

Titleman, P., ed. *Clinical Applications of Bowen Family Systems Theory.* New York: Harworth Press, 1998.

Weiss, R. Cruise Control: Understanding Sex Addiction in Gay Men. Los Angeles: Alyson Books, 2005.

Whybrow, P. C. *American Mania: When More Is Not Enough.* New York: W. W. Norton, 2005.

Index

About the Author

Alexandra Katehakis, M.A., M.F.T., is a nationally recognized expert in the field of sexual disorders. Founder and clinical director of the Center for Healthy Sex (CHS) in Los Angeles, California, she is a certified sex addiction therapist, certified sex therapist, and supervising consultant for the International Institute of Trauma and Addiction Professionals (IITAP). Her articles have been published in the *Journal of Sexual Addiction and Compulsivity, Psychotherapy Networker, Counselor* magazine, and *Family Therapy Magazine.*

Ms. Katehakis and her clinical team at CHS (www.thecenter forhealthysex.com) facilitate the recovery of sexually addicted individuals and assist couples in revitalizing their sex lives. Her area of professional study is applying the latest brain research to the treatment of sexual addiction.

Daily Meditations

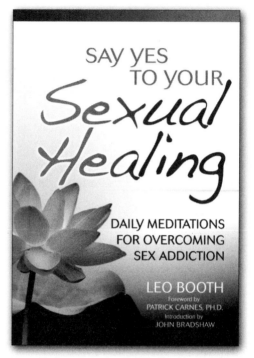

Code # 3787 • Paperback • $12.95

Say Yes to Your Sexual Healing is a daily affirmations book for everyone who has struggled with issues of sex addiction. In *Say Yes to Your Sexual Healing*, Leo Booth offers 365 daily meditations that instill and encourage a healthy and positive outlook on personal hope and healing for each day of the year. Each affirmation emphasizes taking responsibility for one's actions and life and illustrates our daily dance in God's power and how it can lead to happiness, health, satisfaction, and recovery.

Spiritual Journey

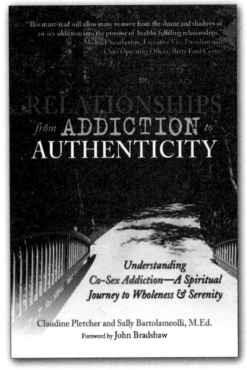

"This must-read will allow many to move from the shame and shadows of co-sex addiction into the promise of healthy fulfilling relationships."
Michael Neatherton, Executive Vice President and Chief Operating Officer, Betty Ford Center

RELATIONSHIPS
from **ADDICTION** *to*
AUTHENTICITY

Understanding
Co-Sex Addiction—A Spiritual
Journey to Wholeness & Serenity

Claudine Pletcher and Sally Bartolameolli, M.Ed.
Foreword by John Bradshaw

Code # 7469 • Paperback • $14.95

Relationships from Addiction to Authenticity is a 12-step spiritual recovery guide written by two survivors of—and experts in—co-sex addiction and is an advocate for restoring the Sacred Feminine Voice that has been muted through co-sex addiction. Sharing their own personal journeys toward renewal and the stories of other women who have tackled the diseases of sex addiction and co-sex addiction, Claudine Pletcher and Sally Bartolameolli, M.Ed., shed light on what you can do to heal the shame that binds you and offer practical advice.

PENGUIN CANADA

THE THRIVE DIET

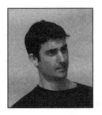

BRENDAN BRAZIER is one of only a few professional athletes in the world whose diet is 100 percent plant based. He's a professional Ironman triathlete, bestselling author on performance nutrition, and the creator of an award-winning line of whole food nutritional products called Vega. He is also the 2003 and 2006 Canadian 50km Ultra Marathon Champion.

Nominated in 2006 for the Manning Innovation Award, Canada's most prestigious award for innovation, Brendan was shortlisted for the formulation of Vega.

In 2006, Brendan also was invited to address US Congress on Capitol Hill, where he spoke of the significant social and economic benefits that could be achieved by improving personal health through better diet. The focus of his talk was to draw attention to the role that food plays in the prevention of most chronic diseases currently plaguing North Americans.

Brendan has become a renowned speaker and sought-after presenter throughout North America, helping individuals and businesses thrive by sharing his dietary stress-busting program, the Thrive Diet.

Brendan lives in Vancouver, BC.